Prescription for WELLNESS

The definitive guide to help you look younger, feel stronger, & live longer

Dr. Ceabert J. Griffith

DISCLAIMER

The ideas, procedures, and recommendations put forth in this book represent only the authors' personal experiences and observations, and are not intended as a substitute for more expert opinions, formulas, and other information regarding a natural anti-aging lifestyle. Readers are advised that each health and wellness expert recommends different and unique approaches to achieving optimal health and longevity. Those who choose to adopt information contained herein are encouraged to confirm its accuracy with their physician.

Because the information in this field is constantly changing, readers should stay informed about new and better techniques and products as they become available. The author and publisher disclaim responsibility for any error, omission, professional disagreement, adverse effect, or unforeseen consequences resulting directly or indirectly from the information and/or products mentioned herein.

The views expressed in this book are the private opinions of the author and do not necessarily reflect the views of the United States Marine Corps, the Department of Defense, or the United States Government.

Library of Congress Cataloging-in-Publication Data

Griffith, Ceabert J
Prescription for Wellness

Bibliography: p.
Include index.
1. Wellness 2. Successful Aging
3. Healthy aging 4. Anti-aging 5. Longevity

ISBN 978-0-615-29000-3
Published by Wellness Press, Tamarac, Florida 33319
To purchase this book, please e-mail: prescriptionforwellness@yahoo.com or visit: http://www.okinawawellness.com

Printed in the United States

To my patients, colleagues and mentors who taught me the art of holistically integrating all the elements of a wellness lifestyle to achieve optimum health and longevity

Foreword

The need to promote health and prevent disease has never been more urgent! Runaway healthcare costs and an escalating disease burden threaten to induce the implosion of the US healthcare system (rather, *sickcare system*). The current $2.5 Trillion healthcare price tag is predicted to go even higher in the coming years—with no logical mechanisms to sustain this unprecedented spending in the out-years. Heart disease, cancer, childhood obesity, and type 2 diabetes among adults and children are some of the exploding health problems that are predicted to impose a decisive blow to the US economy and to the quality of life of every man, woman and child!

It's clearly obvious that the current healthcare system is woefully unprepared to meet the current and future disease burden. Indeed, in its present form, the system is reactive and single-minded. In all fairness, the US healthcare system is one of the best in the world at treating acute illnesses and injuries. But when it comes to chronic diseases such as diabetes, hypertension, osteoarthritis, and dementias—most of which are *preventable*—the current system is impotent and ill-prepared! Further proactive measures are crucially needed to prevent such an epidemic of sickness and injury.

Experts tell us that the fundamental fix for this catastrophe is to teach people how to live healthfully. No question: optimal, comprehensive health—i.e., wellness—is the best antidote to the current crisis.

My friend and colleague, Dr. Ceabert J. Griffith, has delineated the best health promoting/disease preventing plan under one cover that I've ever seen. Indeed, *Prescription for Wellness* shows you the state-of-the-art ways to lower your disease burden and to achieve a long and satisfying life. Bert is a gifted clinician and an exceptional writer. He has his finger on cutting-edge healthcare ideas and knows how to articulate information.

Prescription for Wellness is a synthesis of a cross section of all the latest research from around the world. Bert has nicely integrated this information into a single-source resource guide for you. He effectively discusses the multidimensionality of health and wellness—physical, social, emotional, and spiritual. After reading this book you'll be well equipped to be a co-manager in your healthcare and to adopt the lifestyle strategies that have been shown to help you achieve optimal wellness and longevity. Indeed, this book packs all the information you'll ever need to help you optimize your health and well-being.

I completely endorse Dr. Griffith's wellness prescription because it can potentially help prevent a long list of lifestyle-induced diseases and may help you achieve successful aging. Along with your physician's guidance, this masterpiece can help you look younger, feel stronger and achieve longevity.

Yasuharu Tokuda, M.D., MPH
Clinical Practice Evaluation and Research Center
St. Luke's Life Science Institute
St. Luke's International Hospital
Tokyo, Japan

Acknowledgments

This book was written with the unconditional support of many of my trusted colleagues, mentors, patients, friends, and family members who inspired me to dream big—an indispensable ingredient for success as a writer! When I lost confidence, they conspired to spur me on to the finish line. For this and more, I'm eternally grateful. Many thanks, firstly, to Dr. Yasuharu Tokuda, of the St. Luke's Life Science Institute, St. Luke's International Hospital in Tokyo, Japan who graciously agreed to pen the tone-setting Foreword to this book. Yasu is a true friend, a gifted physician and researcher—despite his youthful age and Harvard University roots (smiles)!

I owe my deepest gratitude to my family who has steadfastly stood by my side through thick and thin, and provided me enormous emotional support and encouragement—free of charge! My wife, Yuko ("Oka-san"), kept the proverbial stiff upper lips and a big smile during my many hours spent researching and writing this book. My two younger children, Kevin and Meg, displayed unparalleled understanding when I announced that this project will steal from our valuable play and vacation time. My two older children, Vanessa and Michael, served as ever present inspirations from afar—I miss them fiercely! My beloved parents, Ceabert and Dora Griffith and my late grandmother, Mrs. Beryl DaCosta, were my inspiration from the very beginning. My brother, Carlos, my sisters, Bernadette and Stacy, and my cousin (sister) Vesta provided badly needed encouragement. I'm very fortunate to have the greatest in-laws in the world: Kinichiro and Masako Kinjo! My brother-in-laws, Satoshi and Tomoji Kinjo, readily applaud my every success.

I'm eternally thankful for Dr. Rod Hooker, my original mentor, who constructively critiqued my very first piece of writing back in 1987. I cherish the special friendship of Mr. Eiichiro Shimabukuro, the Godfather of the 18th Medical Group, and Mr. Morishige Shimabukuro. I thank Dr. Ray Welch, my "bragging buddy" who willingly listens to my incessant whining about my frustrations, dreams, wishes, and (healthy) obsessions. My business buddy (and favorite Kiwi), Glenn McIlvride, has been liberal with his time, counsel and patience. My original Health Promotion partner in crime, Dave Elger, always has wise suggestions for me.

Many thanks to my bosses at Marine Corps Community Services (MCCS), Okinawa, namely, Mr. Steve Pauli, Mr. Rich Milano, and Mr. Ed Hutsell for giving me the best day job a guy can hope for! A big thank you to Ms. Donna LaBarre at the MCCS Semper Fit program office for keeping me out of trouble with the boss! An MCCS shout out to retired SgtMaj Randy Mitchell, USMC, a truly faithful Marine. My staff at the Okinawa Wellness Teaching Center, Ms. Cherryl Castro, Ms. Erin Clemens, Ms. Rika Tazumi, and Mr. Sadaki Higa, is the best in the world!

I deeply appreciate sports medicine physician, Dr. John Biery, for his friendship, professional collaboration, and weekly brainstorming sessions. My special friends and colleagues who directly and indirectly made this project easier include: my crazy neighbor and ultimate prankster, Mike Hertz, who gives freely of his time, patience and comedy relief; my COLA buddy (an inside joke), Jim Allen, PA-C; Ed Wohlschlegels; Josephine Guevara, RN; David Ready, RN; Tara Taylor, RN; Rosalie Weyant, RN; and Art Henriquez.

Since moving to Japan, I've been fortunate to meet and befriend many giants in academia, medicine, and business such as: Mr. Hiroyuki

Nihei (with EM Hotel and Wellness Spa), Dr. Hidemi Todoriki, Dr. Craig Willcox, Dr. David Itokazu, Dr. Minoru Arakaki, Dr. Yasuo Nakahara, Dr. Joe Guarnera, Mr. Yoshi Maizumi, Dr. Moriki Nishihira, Dr. Tomiko Hokama, Dr. Akira Arakaki, Mr. Masamitsu Isa, Mr. Ranjan Sarkar, Dr. Ken Holliday, Dr. Yasuo Nakahara, Associate Professor Liu Asato, Dr. Lyle Allison, and Ms. Michelle Inoya.

I also drew invaluable motivation from supportive folks like Mr. Danny Langton, Ms. Rebecca Langton, LCDR Marc Hawkins, Dr. Joe Martin, and Mr. Ed. Sortino. Finally, my deepest apologies to anyone whose name I neglect to mention!

Dr. Ceabert J. Griffith

How to Read This Book

Prescription for Wellness is organized into seventeen chapters, each one discussing a specific element of wellness. Although each chapter is uniquely focused, each one complements the previous and subsequent chapters, to make for a logical flow of information. I recommend that you read the entire book, beginning with the Foreword and Introduction. However, you may want to first browse the Glossary to familiarize yourself with the terminology appearing in the book and to refer to it thereafter, as needed.

Chapter 1 explains the biomedical principles that govern a wellness-based lifestyle. Chapter 2 examines the diseases linked to poor nutrition and offers practical but simple approaches to eating healthy. In Chapter 3, entitled "Take Dietary Supplements," I discuss the crucial role played by vitamins and minerals in a balanced nutrition regimen, and why most Americans should supplement their diets with these micronutrients. Chapter 4 lists the rationale for engaging in daily physical activity, consequences for physical inertia, and helpful hints on how to get the requisite amount of daily physical activity.

Because overweight and obesity are implicated in so many chronic diseases such as high blood pressure and arthritis, I talk about the importance of maintaining a healthy body weight in Chapter 5. Health experts unanimously agree that quality sleep is the starting point for optimum health and wellness. I, therefore, provide a comprehensive discussion on this subject in Chapters 6. Chapter 7 is devoted to emotional (dis)stress and the litany of health issues it incurs. After reading this chapter, you'll learn nifty tips on how to manage your daily stressors and to stave off one of the most underrated risk factors for poor health and premature death. Chapter 8 highlights one of the most under-recognized downsides of modern living—the lack of healthy social relationships. You'll learn that a fundamental feature of cultures that have achieved optimal health, wellness and longevity is close social ties.

Chapter 9 encourages the reader to adopt a customized spiritual belief system, a strategy that has been shown to promote purpose and meaning in one's life and can help one deal with sorrow and bereavement. Chapters 10 and 11 are about two common vices—tobacco use and alcohol abuse. Using tobacco in any forms is unhealthy and is the single biggest reason for premature death among Americans! Moderate alcohol use promotes health, but alcohol abuse can lead to multiple diseases and early death. Chapter 12 addresses the importance of periodically detoxifying the body, a health promotion strategy that's rapidly gaining traction among Americans.

Traversing the healthcare system can prove to be quite intimidating, especially if you have a chronic medical condition. I believe that healthcare consumers should become savvy in working with healthcare providers. Thus, I included Chapter 13, "Partner with Your Healthcare Providers" to help you learn the nuances of the healthcare industry and how to successfully get the most out of your healthcare experiences. After reading Chapters 14 and 15, which addresses periodic health assessments for women and men, respectively, I hope you'll adopt this strategy as a way to timely identify gaps in your health and take prompt steps to eliminate them.

In Chapter 16, I discuss other healthful practices such as wearing seatbelts when in a car and a helmet when riding a motorcycle, bicycle or skiing. Finally, Chapter 17, the Epilogue, summarizes all the information outlined in *Prescription for Wellness*, and offers a long-term template for achieving a long and healthy lifespan.

The Notes section cites the references used in this book, the comprehensive Glossary of health and wellness terms saves you a lot of time thumbing through a medical dictionary, and the list of suggested readings guides you to additional sources of expert materials. Don't forget the Appendixes, which contain a diet and exercise log and a complete list of health and wellness resources.

Contents

Introduction

"Health is a state of complete physical, mental and social well-being, and not merely the absence of disease or infirmity."
—The World Health Organization, 1948

I'm trained in both natural medicine and family medicine and, for nearly twenty-four years, I've practiced integrative medicine by combining both conventional and complimentary/alternative healing modalities. For the past seven years, I've been a wellness consultant—i.e., a lifestyle coach—guiding patients as they seek to recapture their health. The majority of my current patients are Baby Boomers—members of the celebrated group of nearly 80 million Americans born between 1946 and 1964. Like their politically and economically influential peers, my patients are responsible for the gradual but steady paradigm shift from intervention *sickcare* to prevention, which emphasizes holism and healthy lifestyle choices—i.e., true healthcare.

Central to my current clinical role is helping my patients uncover gaps in their health and develop practical strategies to restore balance (i.e., homeostasis) between the physical, emotional, social and spiritual domains of their lives. This holistic approach to healthcare practice has been the most rewarding of my entire medical career. Evaluating and managing the *whole* person makes more sense than treating isolated pieces of a person's existence. I've watched in awe as my patients transform their lives and delay the onset of age-related diseases by sleeping better, eating healthier, losing weight, jettisoning toxic emotions, and cultivating healthy social relationships.

What I've learn in the past two and one-half decades in medicine is this: Lifestyle choices trump genes when it comes to disease burden, health status, and life expectancy (period)! Moreover, healthy lifestyle choices (e.g., healthy eating and regular physical activity) can avert the need for surgery, chemotherapy, and organ transplant.

Prescription for Wellness reflects my clinical experience (guided by a synthesis of the latest medical research) in helping hundreds of people discover the right mix of therapeutic modalities and lifestyle choices to: reduce chronic pain; lower blood pressure; manage premenstrual syndrome; reduce cholesterol and triglycerides levels; improve digestion; live a stress-free life; beat back insomnia; and achieve numerous other health goals. A wellness-oriented lifestyle has also helped my patients attenuate their risks for heart disease, stroke, diabetes, kidney disease, liver disease, Alzheimer's disease, and various cancers. Many of my patients tell me that, as a result of our consultation, they feel younger and more energetic, sleep better, have improved their social relationships, and have found profound meaning in life. These folks are aging healthfully and are on track to achieve healthy longevity.

GENES, WELLNESS AND HEALTHY AGING

Since the beginning of time, human beings have reluctantly accepted the inevitability of death—despite the immutable fact that the statistical probability of dying is 100%! Two questions have endured throughout human history: *Why do people grow old?* and *What can be done to slow the aging process?* These two questions have been at the core of relentless efforts to find the "fountain of youth" and have been the subject of legends and myths. Indeed, every society in human history has mounted elaborate attempts to uncover the natural course of aging and to stop or delay its onset.

Less than 100 years ago, life expectancy among Americans was a mere 42 years. That President George Washington lived to 67 years old and that Andrew Jackson died at age 78 in 1845 was quite unusual during the 1700s and 1800s. Life expectancy has progressively and dramatically increased to the current 81 years for women and 75 years for men. What accounts for this meteoric almost doubling in life expectancy in such a relatively short time? Is it due to a change in our genetic make-up? Or, is it the result of improvements in healthcare, environmental/public health, and the lifestyle choices we make?

Health experts unanimously agree that human beings have not undergone significant shifts in genetic make-up to account for the dramatic increase in our life expectancy in the past 100 years. What's clear is that healthcare and public health standards have tremendously improved. Moreover, healthy lifestyle choices underscore the success strategies for those who have achieved super-longevity status i.e., the centenarians. In a study that looked at the lifestyle choices of nearly 7,000 individuals between the ages of 45 and 79, seven healthy lifestyle choices—quality sleep, eating breakfast, abstinence from unhealthy snacks, moderate alcohol use, not smoking, a healthy body weight, and regular physical activity—afforded them an extra 14 years of life![1] There's no debating: healthy lifestyle choices (i.e., a adhering to wellness principles) hugely impact our health and the length and quality of our lives.

A "Well" individual enjoys optimal health and well-being in all realms of his life—mind, body, spirit, and social. *Prescription for Wellness*, with its emphasis on the four dimensions of health—the antithesis of the scientific medical model—will show you how to mitigate the top ten chronic diseases in order to support your efforts to achieve optimum health and longevity.

The Four Dimensions of Health and Wellness

Since life is multidimensional, health and wellness, then, must be multidimensional.[2] Indeed, we all have multiple interrelated and inseparable domains of our lives that can be categorized as physical, social, emotional, and spiritual. Some social scientists argue for additional health and wellness domains such as educational, environmental, and cultural well-being. As a clinician, I elect to characterize health and wellness into the four aforementioned categories.

Physical health involves issues of the physical body such as the physical fitness of our bones, muscles, heart, lungs and other organs. Social health has to do with positive interactions and healthy relationships with friends, relatives, co-workers and other acquaintances. If you are emotionally healthy, you have a good self-esteem, positive self-image and balanced mental well-being. The spiritual domain of one's health has to do with finding meaning, purpose and value in one's life through awareness and acknowledgement of a higher power or being in the universe. Prayer, meditation, and other spiritually-based rituals all contribute to spiritual wellness.

Wellness is therefore a state of total harmony of your inner self, external life, and the universe at large. In fact, you're healthier when each of your four domains is taken care of and they interdependently converge. For example, when an individual is physically healthy, it's easier for him to: have a sense of self-efficacy; have a positive outlook on life; realize a sense of purpose in life; and form healthy relationships. Weaving these four health domains together is what health and wellness is all about.

Unfortunately, allopathic physicians are not trained to recognize the inseparable nature of these four health domains. In fact, allopathic medicine largely zeros in on the physical and mental health of patients and ignores patients' social and spiritual domains. A litany of research in the past couple of decades clearly shows that humans heal faster, are happier, and achieve healthy longevity when all four domains of their existence are recognized and cultivated. *Prescription for Wellness* will recommend simple but practical ways to achieve optimal levels of function within each of these domains, and show you how to weave together these domains to experience a high level of well-being, slow the aging process, and possibly achieve longevity.

A WELLNESS LIFESTYLE: MYTHS AND FACTS

A glaring shortfall of conventional medicine is its failure to recognize and/or articulate the fact that optimal health and wellness is well within the reach of most people. The current US healthcare system is virtually focused on treating diseases and spectacularly less interested in promoting health and preventing diseases. As a result, the average person isn't aware of the steps he can take to optimize his health and well-being. Let's now examine some commonly held myths regarding health and wellness and replace them with evidence-based facts:

***MYTH*: "I can accept the physical, emotional and social domains of wellness, but the spiritual domain makes me uneasy. I'm not religious and don't believe in ghosts."**

***FACT*:** The spiritual domain of wellness is one of the hardest to explain to Americans, mostly because Western cultures don't emphasize the spiritual side of human existence—except within the context of religion. However, spirituality doesn't necessarily refer to religion or religious practices; an individual can be spiritual without being religious, and vice versa. As you'll learn in Chapter 9, spiritual health can be achieved through many secular philosophies and practices such as yoga, music and meditation. Some people chose religion, but there are plenty of options to satisfy every taste and desire. Spirituality forms the basis by which we define our deepest purpose in life. Dr. Wayne Dwyer, one of the most celebrated modern-day U.S. philosophers, believes that humans are fundamentally spiritual beings having human experiences rather than the other way around.

***MYTH*: "Genetic endowment is the final arbiter of an individual's health and wellness. Why try to adopt healthy behaviors when my inherited propensity will determine the level of health, wellness, and lifespan I can achieve?"**

FACT: This is simply not true. A large body of research in the past few decades reveals that, while genetic endowment plays a major role in someone's health, wellness and longevity status, lifestyle choices are most important. For example, twin studies have shown that identical twin (with identical genome) who are raised separately develop different health profiles and life expectancies. "Our faulty genes load the gun; our lifestyle pulls the trigger" was coined by pioneering diabetic specialist, the late Dr. Elliot Joslin, and is now a common adage in the natural medicine world. Our DNA doesn't seal our destiny. Therefore, the premise of total wellness is that good health and longevity have more to do with individual lifestyle choices and less to do with genetics.

Genetically-connected diseases that are hugely influenced by lifestyle choices include high blood pressure (or hypertension), type 2 diabetes, heart disease, stroke, and osteoporosis. We know, for example, that hypertension runs in families and that a number of genes have been connected to its development. However, many people without a family history of hypertension develop the condition. Conversely, many people have normal blood pressure despite having both parents with chronically elevated blood pressure. If you examine the risk factors for hypertension, the majority of them are lifestyle-related: excessive psychological stress; tobacco use; overweight and obesity; physical inactivity; and excessive intake of sodium and alcohol. Genetic endowment is not the final arbiter of an individual's health, wellness, and life span.

MYTH: **"With so many life challenges facing people everyday (e.g., psychological stress at work and at home), it is impossible to achieve optimal wellness and slow the aging process."**

FACT: There is no question that there are enduring challenges to each domain of wellness but, in most cases, these challenges can be overcome. For example, as you'll learn in Chapter 7, stress is a ubiquitous reality of daily life, but there are very effective ways of minimizing its effects. Indeed, perception is a major element of what makes an event or experience stressful. Recognizing this will go a long way in taking the steam out of a stressful situation. Speaking of stress—reducing stress can minimize physical pain, improve cognitive function, and help foster a generally-positive attitude, factors that can facilitate good health and wellness.

***MYTH*: "A wellness-based lifestyle is a luxury, available only to the rich and famous, not to us poor folks."**

***FACT*:** This is false. Wellness is available to virtually everyone, regardless of race, gender, socioeconomic status, religion, or any other demographic characteristic. As you'll come to understand while reading this book, some acute and most chronic illnesses can be traced to physical, emotional, social, or spiritual dysfunction. The ability to restore these functions is within the reach of just about everyone. For example, type 2 diabetes and hypertension can be effectively held in check by engaging in 30 minutes of physical activity each day—not a terribly expensive proposition for most people.

***MYTH*: "The recalcitrant nature of some chronic diseases effectively precludes the achievement of health and wellness."**

***FACT*:** I agree that some diseases such as asthma are incurable and the best you can hope for is disease palliation and functional health. However, this is true in relatively few cases. Most chronic disease are connected to poor nutrition, physical inactivity, the use of tobacco products, excessive alcohol consumption and excessive stress—factors all related to lifestyle choices. Making healthy lifestyle choices can eliminate or attenuate most diseases that can get in the way of achieving optimal health and wellness. For example, numerous studies have demonstrated that eating a so-called Mediterranean Diet (see Chapter 2) imparts an impressive list of health benefits: lowered risk of heart disease; reduced risk for certain cancers; lowered cholesterol levels; reduced inflammation; and improved health of the inner lining of blood vessels.

HOW THIS BOOK CAN HELP YOU

Why is this wellness book different from others on the market today? Is this another so-called "me too" book that repackages the same old information? I believe that you'll find that, unlike other wellness books, this primer nicely achieves dual goals: firstly, it educates the reader about *all* the elements of good health and wellness; and, secondly, it shows the reader how to integrate these insights and practices into his or her daily life to achieve successful aging and, possibly, longevity. I do this by: using simple prose to explain what wellness is and isn't to dispel the many myths about its achievement; describing practical strategies for adopting each wellness piece; and delineating various options for closing gaps in your health status that might preclude the achievement of high-level wellness.

I also discuss the multi-dimensionality of a wellness-centric lifestyle. Most wellness books on the market deal with only a single dimension of health strategies such as plastic surgery, which gives the *appearance* of healthy aging or hormonal replacement therapy, which produces artificial *feelings* of youth and vitality. Experts such as Dr. Andrew Weil and Dr. Ray Sahelian will tell you that the process of healthy aging is inexorably multi-dimensional and largely natural! The human body has an unbelievable capacity to heal itself and to stay youthful and energetic through healthy lifestyle choices.

In the end, *Prescription for Wellness* will help make you a healthier winner! This book can potentially help you:

- Boost your brainpower
- Augment your energy level

- Reduce mental stress
- Strengthen your immune function
- Improve your flexibility
- Lose weight
- Understand the innate wisdom of your body
- Bolster overall health
- Achieve healthy aging and longevity

I hope that this book, by laying out a simple roadmap for you (based on cutting-edge research), will serve as a single source manual that will help expand your health and wellness knowledge. I hope this knowledge will then motivate you to achieve the determination and commitment needed to make healthy lifestyle choices. I also hope that this knowledge will empower you to enter into meaningful collaboration with your physician, physician assistant/associate, nurse, nurse practitioner, optometrist, and other members of your health care team to avoid the horrific consequences of chronic—but *preventable*—diseases that plague an increasingly large portion of the American population.

WHAT YOU CAN DO TO HELP YOURSELF

Ultimately, the adoption of healthy lifestyle choices rests squarely on your shoulders. Only you—not your doctor or nurse—can control how much sodium and alcohol you consume, how well you manage your daily stressors, or how well you adhere to an exercise program. I'm in no way suggesting that you walk out on your healthcare team; rather, I encourage you to form a more collegial relationship with your family doctor, dietitian, optometrist, personal trainer and other fitness and health professionals. With help and support from your team of health and fitness experts supplemented by the information in this book, you'll be well on your way to developing the skill, motivation, and commitment needed to live a wellness-oriented life. You're in far more control of your health than you realize. The ball is in your court!

Chapter 1

Anatomy of a Wellness Lifestyle

"Life is not merely to be alive, but to be well."
—Marcus Valerius Martial
Roman Poet, 38-104 AD

The importance of a wellness lifestyle has been recognized for centuries. In this chapter, I'll provide an overview of a wellness-centric lifestyle, which will set the stage for an in-depth discussion of each wellness element in subsequent chapters. It's important to point out that wellness is a dynamic way of living that aims to achieve optimum physical, social, emotional, and spiritual health.

What does it take to achieve wellness? What are the barriers to a wellness lifestyle and how to overcome these challenges? Let's examine the short answers to these questions.

ROADMAP TO A WELLNESS LIFESTYLE

I happen to believe that growing old is inevitable but that the rate of aging is optional and modifiable. How well—or poorly—we age is, in large measure, due to the manner in which we elect to live. But this isn't just my opinion. In a seminal book on aging, Drs. Rowe and Kahn showed that the biology of the aging process is dominated by non-genetic influences such as level of physical activity, nutrition choices, and psychological health and social connectedness.[1] They estimated that genetic endowment exerts only about a 30 percent influence on how we age!

This gene/lifestyle observation was made among the centenarians of Okinawa, Japan and discussed eloquently in the New York Times bestselling book *The Okinawa Program* by researchers, Drs. Bradley Willcox, Craig Willcox, and Makoto Suzuki.[2] More recently, Dan Buettner, an explorer and documentary producer, documented the robust lifestyle strategies of the world's longest lived people in his bestselling book, *The Blue Zones*.[3] The central theme of these masterpieces is that healthy aging is a daily habit that most people can develop!

Today, many prominent gerontologists and longevity experts share Drs. Rowe's and Kahn's belief that lifestyle factors should be exploited as the best healthy aging strategies. These include: good nutrition; the use of selected dietary supplements for some; daily physical activity for all; maintaining a healthy weight; and getting quality sleep. Other healthy aging strategies include: managing excessive stress; having good social connections; adopting a spiritual belief system; refraining from using tobacco products; and using alcohol in moderation.

Successful aging also involves detoxification for optimal health; undergoing periodic health evaluations; forming a strategic alliance with your healthcare team; limiting sun exposure; and wearing protective devices such as seatbelts and a bicycle helmet. *Prescription for Wellness* is a roadmap to adopting these evidence-based, age-defying strategies.

Let's briefly examine the evidence for each of these lifestyle factors before delving into each one more deeply in subsequent chapters.

Healthy Nutrition Practices

That *food is medicine* is not a cute slogan but an undeniable fact recognized as far back in time as 370 B.C. by Hippocrates, the father of modern medicine. In the past 100 years, our quest for technological medicine caused us to lose sight of the fact that the foods we eat can protect our DNA and help our body's innate healing abilities. That Okinawa, the beautiful Archipelagos south of the main Japanese island, is home to one of the highest concentration of centenarians on earth is largely due to the plant- and fish-based diet of the older Okinawans. In their New York Times bestselling book *The Okinawa Diet*

Plan, Drs. Makoto Suzuki, Craig Willcox, and Bradley Willcox superbly connects the dietary (and other) factors with the achievement of healthy longevity among older Okinawans. In Chapter 2, I discuss anti-aging nutrition practices in detail.

Dietary Supplements

The best way to get micronutrients is via whole foods. However, most Americans fail to get the requisite number of fruits and vegetables in their diet, leaving a large percent of the population deficient in vitamins, minerals, phytonutrients, and other nutrients needed to drive virtually all biochemical processes in the body. Therefore, dietary supplements are recommended to fill nutrition gaps for individuals who fail to get enough micronutrients from whole foods. In Chapter 3, I'll examine the merits of taking daily nutritional supplements for most people.

Daily Physical Activity

The human body was made to be moved. One of the surest anti-aging strategies is physical activity. As I discuss in Chapter 4, people who are physically active enjoy better health and a higher quality of life, and they live longer than their inactive peers. Indeed, if exercise were a pill, it would be the most popular pill ever invented as it would fix most chronic diseases, and the inventor would be the world's first mega-trillionaire! Get moving and you'll instantly start to slow the velocity with which you age by keeping age-related diseases at bay.

Maintain a Healthy Weight

An unhealthy body mass index (BMI) is an independent risk factor for a long list of diseases such as diabetes, osteoarthritis, cancer and high blood pressure. I delineate the evidence of this in Chapter 5 and discuss nifty and painless ways to maintain a healthy BMI.

Quality Sleep

Poor quality sleep can make you sick and contribute to your early demise. As I discuss in Chapter 6, the epidemic of poor quantity and quality of sleep experienced by most Americans is a major contributor to obesity, cognitive impairment, heart disease and many other 21st-century health problems. *"Sleep your way to good health"* is not a hyperbole; it's reality.

Stress Management

Stress, the ubiquitous villain that permeates the lives of most Americans, is the backdrop of most of the top 10 killers of Americans today. The negative effects of this stealth killer can't be over exaggerated. Fortunately, excessive stress can be greatly minimized if you are committed to doing so. Chapter 7 will inspire you to follow simple but effective stress managing techniques in your daily life.

Good Social Connections

When life's crises hit—as they inevitably will—it's nice to have close friends and relatives to turn to for support. You're almost always better able to weather setbacks with the help of a network of staunch well-wishers. Chapter 8 shows you how.

A Spiritual Belief System

Western cultures are more and more beginning to understand that spirituality is an indispensable part of health and wellness. Spiritual awareness involves a wide spectrum of practices that range from simple meditation to organized religion and everything in between. As Chapter 9 discusses, spiritual groundedness can help you find profound meaning in life and can help deal with bereavement and sorrow.

Don't Use Tobacco

Chapter 10 examines the most preventable cause of death among Americans—tobacco usage. If you use tobacco, you should stop as soon as you can and if you don't use tobacco you shouldn't start. It's a most difficult habit to break but, with perseverance, even to most committed tobacco user can kick the habit! I'll fill you in on the most effective strategies for parting company with this dangerous product.

Limited Alcohol Use

Alcohol is a double-edge sword; it's both good and bad for you. You may have read or heard of the health-imparting properties of small amounts of red wine, but the dangers imposed by using too much of this ancient product will send you to an early grave. In Chapter 11, I'll review the scientific literature on the health benefits of moderate alcohol use, describe the litany of diseases alcohol abuse can incur, and offer up some ways to achieve sobriety and to stay that way.

Detoxification for Optimal Health

It's becoming clearer that despite the heroic efforts of the body's own detoxification system, toxic metabolites accumulate in the body due to environmental pollution, emotional stress, chronic inflammation, and long-term diseases. These toxins stifle cell and organ function making it more difficult for the body to make energy, lose weight, get quality sleep, manage stress, and perform myriad other physiological functions. In Chapter 12, I recommend a system for periodically cleansing the body and restoring optimum cell and organ function.

Working with your Healthcare Team

That 45 million Americans are uninsured and millions more underinsured is a sad testimony to our flawed system of national priorities.

Every person should have access to a team of healthcare professionals to help guide and monitor his or her health status. Currently, *sickness care* is a sacred cash cow that benefits too many people and organizations that are not willing to support universal healthcare for Americans. I'll describe the inner workings of our current sickness care system in Chapter 13 and recommend strategies for working collegially with members of your care team to make a less-than-optimal system more accessible and responsive to your healthcare needs.

Periodic Health Evaluations

Knowing your health status is as relevant as knowing your financial status. We should all undergo periodic physical examinations to quantify our health and identify potential life-shortening diseases. Having a health "report card" can motivate you to improve your health; you'll be more committed to work on the health areas where you score Cs, Ds, and Fs. Check out Chapters 14 and 15.

Other Wellness Strategies

Four safety issues round out my healthy aging strategies: limiting excessive sun exposure; wearing seatbelts; wearing bicycle and motorcycle helmets; and minimizing the use of cell phones. Like alcohol, sun exposure is a double-edged sword: a little is good for you; too much is bad for you. Seatbelts do save lives as do safety helmets. Electromagnetic radiation emitted by cell phones appears to negatively impact brain health. As I discuss in Chapter 16, adhering to these safety practices is just as important as adhering to a low saturated fat diet.

BARRIERS TO A WELLNESS LIFESTYLE

In my clinical practice, I'm amazed by the huge gap between *knowledge* and *action* among some of my patients. The vast majority of my patients are quite knowledgeable and savvy about what it takes to live healthfully and well. Virtually no one comes into my office saying "I didn't know that exercise is good for you!" Everyone knows that high blood cholesterol can clog arteries, which can then lead to a heart attack or stroke. All of my patients know that extra body weight is very unhealthy and can lead to osteoarthritis, diabetes, and some types of cancers.

Unfortunately, a strong knowledge base doesn't always spur a person into action. Without my coaching, few of my patients would spontaneously act on their knowledge. In fact, the crux of my practice is to bridge the gap between *Wellness Knowledge* and *Wellness Action*; getting my patients to apply what they already know to their daily lives. I do this by exploring the barriers that impede their best efforts to implement and/or sustain their lifestyle plan. The most common barriers include lack of motivation, improper prioritization, stress, anxiety, depression, procrastination, and poor time management. Therefore, I resort to inspiring them to start living a wellness lifestyle by creatively jumping over or going around the hurdles that stand between them and optimal health and wellness.

These barriers are many and include: lack of motivation, flawed prioritization, excessive stress (distress), anxiety, depression, procrastination, and poor time management. Let's now examine each one of these hurdles:

Lack of Motivation

I believe that one has to have a *motive* to become motivated. When it comes to health and wellness, the best motive is to want to maintain an optimal quality of life—throughout one's lifespan. What is optimal quality of life? How can the desire for optimal quality of life motivate you to adopt healthy practices?

I have never met anyone who hoped for an early demise. Indeed, a most enduring wish of humans is to live healthy and for a long time. Unfortunately, many people believe that a long, healthy life is a dream for a chosen few with robust genetic endowment. Research in the past few decades has shown that genetic endowment notwithstanding, our health depends on the lifestyle we chose for ourselves. As I mentioned in the Introduction, "Our faulty genes load the gun; our lifestyle pulls the trigger" was coined by pioneering diabetic specialist the late Dr. Elliot Joslin, and is now a common adage in the natural medicine world. It's crystal clear that our DNA doesn't seal our destiny; good health and longevity have more to do with individual lifestyle choices and less to do with genetics.

Flawed Prioritization

A good plan is virtually useless if your priorities are out of place. You should assign levels of importance to your various obligations. As Stephen Covey, author of *The 7 Habits of Highly Effective People* states, you must fundamentally know your "big rocks" and your "small rocks" in life. Get in the habit of taking care of your big rocks before taking care of your small rocks. Decide what's most important in your life (hopefully good health is at the top of your list) and take care of the most important things first. Indeed, the things that matter least must never take priority over the things that matter most!

Excessive Stress

I believe that chronic and excessive stress is *the* most underrated and unrecognized risk factor for a long list of diseases, including heart disease, stroke, diabetes, high blood pressure, and some cancers. Unlike blood pressure and cholesterol level, we cannot objectively measure stress, so it's relegated to subjective assessment. Because we live very busy lives, we ignore the physiological effects of excessive stress. Therefore, stress gets a free pass. Don't fall for this tendency—recognize the ill-effects of emotional distress and learn ways to manage this ubiquitous killer (see Chapter 7).

Anxiety

Anxiety robs you of your energy, creativity, and motivation. When you are anxious, it's difficult to envision high possibilities. Instead, you're constantly worrying about failures and setbacks. Your unconscious and conscious minds join forces to stymie all of your efforts to move forward in life. Anxiety is truly a major league barrier to wellness.

Depression

Depression can imprison the most well-intentioned person. Like anxiety, depression forms an immovable barrier to new heights. Depression can be insidious and lethal—you should see your doctor promptly for an evaluation and management plan.

Procrastination

Procrastination is a virulent habit that's at the root of most cases of failure to succeed. And the root cause of procrastination is the fear of failure. The best resource I've ever reviewed on how to stop procrastinating is a wonderfully written little book entitled *Eat that Frog* by best-selling author, Brian Tracy. Every procrastinator should purchase this book and read it as many times as it takes to start practicing Brain Tracy's great recommendations.

Poor Time Management

How you manage your time can be the difference between a successful and an unsuccessful life. Allocating how you spend your time is crucial to achieving any personal or professional goal. Here again, I recommend Brain Tracy's bestselling book, *Eat that Frog.*

KNOCKING DOWN WELLNESS BARRIERS

With the right motive and plan, most people are able to bridge the gap between knowledge and action. I have encountered very few people who are downright ill-equipped to start a walking program, begin managing their stress, or start eating vegetables. Here's what it takes to knock down the barriers to a wellness lifestyle:

Quantify the Importance of your Health

We all consciously and unconsciously prioritize our daily behaviors. Our prioritization is based on perceived need and perceived threat. We place work at a higher level of priority over play because of the need to earn a living to fund daily obligations. Unfortunately, most people fail to place healthy behaviors (e.g., play) at the top of their priority list. I believe that this is due to a lack of perceived short-term threat. In other words, there're no terrible immediate consequences for eating three unhealthy meals today! Even when our poor health behavior incurs a short-term consequence—e.g., heartburn from eating spicy foods right before bedtime—there are rapid fixes for our transgressions (e.g., antacid that take away the acute symptoms in less than 30 minutes).

The first order of business for knocking down the barriers to a wellness lifestyle is to decide deeply and strongly where your health and well-being stack up with the rest of the issues in your life. Is your health as important as work? Does your health mean more to you than the brief pleasure derived from eating a high-fat meal?

In my nearly 24 years of medical practice, virtually all of my patients, when asked, espouse that their health and well-being was the most important resource in their lives. Unfortunately, only a handful ever exhibit the behavior supporting their public pronouncement!

Develop a SMART Wellness Lifestyle Plan

Behavioral specialists will tell you that plans involving lifestyle changes are difficult to implement. After all, what you are trying to change are old habits—very deeply ingrained behaviors. To ensure success, you should develop a Wellness Lifestyle Plan that is: specific, measurable, achievable, realistic, and time-bound, and can be remembered using the acronym, SMART. These five elements can also function as a litmus test when you re-evaluate your Wellness Lifestyle Plan.

You should also write down your plan on paper. This cements your goals in your mind and subconscious and gives life and true meaning to your plan.

Let's now look at each piece of a SMART Wellness Lifestyle Plan:

Specific. You stand a better chance of achieving success with your Wellness Lifestyle Plan if your goals are as specific as possible. They should be straightforward and should clearly state what it is you hope to accomplish. Having specific goals helps you focus your efforts on the things you need to do to succeed. Specific goals represent the *who, what, where, why, when, how* of your Wellness Lifestyle Plan. An example of a specific goal would be: "Walk from 6:30 am to 7:30 am, on Mondays, Wednesdays, and Fridays of each week."

Measurable. You should be able to measure your progress as you work towards your goals. As the old business saying go: *if you can't measure it, you can't manage it*. For example, a goal "to eat healthier" isn't measurable. A measurable goal is "to eat 5 servings of vegetables at lunch and 5 servings at dinner, daily, by Thanksgiving." Come Thanksgiving, if you're eating only six servings of vegetables a day you haven't achieved your goal and have to re-double your efforts. Measurable goals allow you to experience the exhilaration of progress that serves to motivate you to continue your efforts.

Achievable. Your goals should be realistically attainable. If you are 5' 8" and 250 pounds at age 55, it will be very difficult—highly unlikely—to get down to the 130 pounds you were at age 25. A wellness plan with this unattainable goal is doomed from the start. I'd suggest you select a more realistic and achievable goal weight—say, a goal weight of 155 pounds. Many people fail to succeed because they strive for fundamentally unattainable goals—and fail!

Realistic. Your goals must be realistic and doable. This will arm you with the willingness and ability to pursue your goals. For example, a wellness goal "to never again eat sweets" is unrealistic for most people. A more realistic goal is "to eat sweets no more than once weekly—no more than 52 times a year."

Time-bound. You must decide on specific timelines for your goals. Otherwise, you'll be locked in a viscous cycle of procrastination and stagnation. By setting deadlines, you'd have a specific date to work towards. Be sure to set sensible deadlines or risk not taking them seriously.

Execute your Wellness Lifestyle Plan

Like any good plan, a healthy aging lifestyle plan should be executed with precision and clarity. The SMART framework will provide you a tangible roadmap from which to execute your plan.

Re-evaluate your Wellness Lifestyle Plan

The fundamental trick to a successfully executable wellness plan is periodic re-evaluation and modification. Re-looking at your plan helps you to objectively see where you fall short and what it is you need to do the tweak your efforts. With your new modification in mind you can develop a new self-image, complete with renewed motivation, conviction, and confidence!

IN SUMMARY

- A successful wellness lifestyle is characterized by: daily physical activity; a healthy weight; quality sleep; stress management; good social connection; a solid spiritual belief system; abstinence from tobacco; limited alcohol intake; periodic health evaluations; and working with your healthcare team. Other strategies include limited sun exposure, wearing seatbelts, and wearing a bicycle helmet.
- A lack of knowledge, improper prioritization, stress, anxiety, depression, procrastination, and poor time management can stymie your best efforts to implement and sustain a wellness plan.
- Effective strategies for knocking down barriers to your wellness plan include: quantifying the importance of your health; developing a SMART Wellness Lifestyle Plan that's specific, measurable, achievable, relevant, and time bound; executing your plan; and periodically re-evaluating your plan.

Chapter 2

Eat Healthfully

"Of the ten leading causes of death in the United States, four, including the top three, are associated with dietary excesses: coronary heart disease, some types of cancer, stroke, and non-insulin-dependent diabetes mellitus. Together these conditions account for nearly two-thirds of the deaths each year in the United States. "

—Elizabeth Frazao, *"The High Cost of Poor Diets"*
USDA Food Review

Like Elizabeth Frazao, many health experts, such as Dr. Andrew Weil of the University of Arizona, School of Medicine, believe that there is a nutritional basis for the vast majority of chronic diseases that currently plague Americans. As a matter of fact, a very large body of research implicates poor nutrition in the development of diabetes, high blood pressure, heart disease, stroke, osteoporosis, some forms of arthritis, and some types of cancers. Preliminary evidence indicts unhealthy nutrition practices as a contributing factor in the development of Alzheimer's disease and other dementias.

Good nutrition is one of the indispensable cornerstones of good health and wellness, healthy aging, and disease prevention—akin to good medicine. But this isn't a modern-day discovery. Hippocrates, the father of medicine, said over two millenniums ago: "Let food be thy medicine and thy medicine be thy food."

Today, the definition of good nutrition seems to be a moving target for many people. The average person is desperately confused by the conflicting opinions and scientific information out there. As Michael Pollan brilliantly discusses in his bestselling book *In Defense of Food*, nutrition in America has undergone radical shifts in definition and subjected to political and other non-scientific influences.[1] For example, we changed the discourse from whole foods to individual nutrients to accommodate the industrialization of *food-like* products. What we now call food is merely nutrients scientifically engineered to increase food manufacturers' profit margins.

So, what's good nutrition? What does it mean to eat healthfully? Well, in a capsule, good nutrition is eating nutrient-dense foods—those packing the most vitamins, minerals, macronutrients, phytochemicals, and fiber for the fewest number of calories. This means fresh, high-quality, organic, unprocessed, whole foods. Let's now look at the components of good nutrition and explore creative ways to adopt healthy eating habits.

COMPONENTS OF GOOD NUTRITION

One of the great paradoxes of American life in the 21st century is that despite the abundance of food, we are terribly undernourished. Sadly, the root of our undernourishment has to do with our food supply and the way we accept the packaging of our food. The human body has evolved to subsist on natural foods. In fact, the optimum human diet is plant-based.

In the past four or five decades, our food supply has become toxic and unhealthy. In the name of science, we've engineered a food supply characterized by polysyllabic chemicals geared to ensure a shelf life of 2 to 15 years! And we've all accepted this abominable practice; we don't care that the "food" we eat today was manufactured and put in a can over three years ago along with preservatives, artificial coloring, trans-fats and salt! We also have no qualms about imbibing on cheap, "fast-food" invariably loaded with unhealthy fats, calories, sugars, and salt.

As informed consumers, how can we charter a smart course of healthy eating? What are the elements of good nutrition practices? Based on a synthesis of current scientific evidence, the basics of a wellness-centric and longevity-supporting nutrition practices are:

- "Don't eat anything your great-grandmother wouldn't recognize as food," advises Michael Pollan.[1]
- Consume three balanced meals plus three healthy snacks each day.
- Cut your current portion size by 10 percent. (Later in this section, I'll discuss the amount of calories you should consume).
- Get 5 to 10 servings of vegetables and fruits daily. Be sure to consume a variety because each one has its own nutrient profile. Minimize fruits because of their high sugar content. Vegetables contain disease-fighting phytochemicals, which are a group of 10,000 plant-derived nutrients that have health promoting and disease preventing properties.
- Minimize your intake of saturated and the so-called trans-fats. Get adequate amounts of healthy fats from olive oil.
- Eat only low-calorie protein from fish, chicken, legumes (beans), nuts, seeds, and soy products. Minimize animal protein.
- Eat only complex carbohydrates.
- Minimize sodium intake.
- Reduce caffeine intake.
- Get adequate amounts of calcium, magnesium, and potassium, preferably from whole foods.
- Avoid dining out, if possible; this is one of the banes of unhealthy eating!

Appropriate Amount of Calories

An important component to good nutrition is adherence to the appropriate caloric intake for your age, gender, body mass index and your daily activities. As we age, our caloric requirements lessen. A 30 year-old person, for instance, has a higher caloric need than a 60 year-old. The following represents the approximate basal caloric needs per day based on age, during different stages of life:

- Newborns require 22 cal/lb of body weight
- Toddlers require 26 cal/lb of body weight
- Teenagers require 18 cal/lb of *ideal* body weight
- 30 year-olds require 13 cal/lb of *ideal* body weight
- 45 year-olds require 12 cal/lb of *idea*l body weight
- 60 year-olds require 10 cal/lb of *idea*l body weight

The above is a general estimate of caloric requirements per day. Because people with certain health conditions may have a more precise caloric needs, you should check with your doctor or nutritionist to help you calculate your exact calories requirement.

Solid research in the past few decades suggests that the amount of calories we consume can influence our lifespan. In a scientific paper published in 2007 in *Annals of the New York Academy of Sciences*, scientists studying exceptional longevity among Okinawans (the southern-most Japanese State, where I currently live) found that calorie restriction helps reduce age-related diseases and extend lifespan. The Okinawans have a famous saying *Hara Hachi Bu* which translates into eating up to the point where you are 80 percent full.

Reduced caloric intake results in positive biomarkers that prevent the accumulation of toxic metabolites in the body. Indeed, caloric restriction can lower blood pressure, cholesterol levels, and fasting blood sugar levels, and supports a healthy immune system, proving that less is sometimes better.

How to reduce your daily calories? Obviously, this is a change that will be difficult to implement—especially if you currently consume a diet very high in calories. Check with your healthcare provider before drastically reducing your calories as there is a potential for untoward side effects, such as low blood sugar. However you decide to approach calorie restriction, you should do it gradually and be guided by your body's response to the new way of eating. Strive for nutrient-dense foods and promptly report any undue health effects to your healthcare provider.

Healthy Fats

Fats add taste to foods, serve as long-term energy stores, transport fat-soluble vitamins (i.e., vitamins A, D, E and K), form the membrane of cells, and serve numerous other health functions. The adult brain is 60 percent fat and infants need a good supply of fat for brain development. Hence, fat is an indispensible macronutrient.

Currently, there is a fierce debate among health experts about the role of fats in health and disease. The consensus is that there are "healthy" and "unhealthy" fats, and that we should aim for a higher percentage of healthy fats in our diet. The American Heart Association recommends that people consume no more than 30 percent of their total daily calories in fat, of which no more than 10 percent should be from the saturated variety.

There are three types of fats: saturated, polyunsaturated, and monounsaturated. Saturated fats—generally, those that are solid at room temperature—have been shown to increase LDL or bad cholesterol while lowering HDL or good cholesterol in the blood, leading to clogged arteries and cardiovascular disease. Saturated fats are found mainly in animal foods, including meat, poultry skin, whole milk, butter, and cheese. Palm and coconut oils are 50 percent and 85 percent saturated fats, respectively.

It's important to remember that foods touted as fat-free are not *exactly* free of fat. The Food and Drug Administration (FDA) permits food manufacturers to use the following terminology on food and drug labels when referring to fat content:

- Fat free: Contains less than 0.5 g of fat per serving.
- Reduced fat: Contains at least 25 percent less fat than normally found in comparable foods.
- Light: Contains half the fat or one-third the calories normally found in comparable foods.
- Low fat: Contains less fat without having to quantify the amount, but generally no more than 3 gm of fat per serving.

Polyunsaturated fats are safer than saturated fats but still pose some health risks. These fats are liquid at room temperature. Sources of these fats include vegetable oils (e.g., corn, safflower, and sunflower oils), margarine, shortening, mayonnaise, and salad dressing.

Monounsaturated fats are the safest type of fat. It's felt to lower LDL cholesterol while preserving HDL cholesterol, referred to as "good" or "protective" cholesterol because it removes artery-clogging cholesterol and other materials from the blood stream. Monounsaturated fat is found mainly in a variety of oils, including macadamia nut, olive, avocado, grape seed, canola, and fish oil. Omega-3 fats—found in salmon, tuna, and other cold-water fish—reduce inflammation, lessen PMS, and regulate cardiovascular, nervous, reproductive and immune systems. You should take a daily supplement of 1000-3000 mg.

Trans-fats or hydrogenated fats are manufactured by adding hydrogen to vegetable oil—a process referred to as hydrogenation. Trans-fats stabilize the flavor of foods and increase their shelf-life. You should avoid trans-fats at all cost as they are worse than saturated fats and have been shown to be major contributors to heart disease and stroke by raising LDL cholesterol and lowering HDL cholesterol. New York City and other State and local jurisdictions have enacted laws banning the use of these deadly fats.

Foods and food-like products that contain trans-fats include: vegetable shortenings, margarine, mayonnaise, bacon, sausage, hot dogs, French fries, microwave popcorn, potato chips, cheese crackers, saltine crackers, cakes, doughnuts, pound cake, Danish pastry, white bread, dinner rolls, corn muffins, cookies, and chocolate bars.

Healthy Carbohydrates

Carbohydrates are a source of quick energy. These nutrients also help build cell membrane. Carbohydrates come in two distinct forms: simple (e.g., table sugar and white bread) and complex (e.g., beans and whole-grain bread). You should stay away from simple carbohydrates because they digest quickly and spike blood sugar levels, which elicit a concomitant insulin spike. Chronic insulin spikes have been linked to the development of type 2 diabetes, hypertension, coronary artery disease, stroke, and some cancers.

On the other hand, complex carbohydrates have low-glycemic indices—i.e., they take a longer time to digest and don't attract a rapid spike in blood insulin levels. Furthermore, complex carbohydrates contain more vitamins, minerals, phytonutrients and other nutrients compared to simple carbohydrates. You should aim for low-glycemic, complex carbs such as oatmeal, cereals, brown rice, and vegetables.

Fiber. A most important indigestible carbohydrate is fiber (also referred to as "roughage" or "bulk"). Lacking in calories, vitamins and minerals, fiber exists in two forms: soluble fiber, which dissolves in water to form a gel-like substance; and insoluble fiber, which can't dissolve in water, but adds bulk to the stool. Sources of soluble fiber include legumes (beans, lentils, and peas), oats and berries. Nuts, seeds, whole grains, and whole wheat provide insoluble fiber.

Popularized in the 1970s by British Surgeon and medical researcher, Dr. Denis Burkitt, fiber is now recognized as a "Super Food." Indeed, this rock star of nutrients is the favorite of nutritionists, gastroenterologists, cardiologists, and diabetologists. Working in Africa where the dietary fiber intake of Africans is relatively high compared to Europeans, Dr. Burkitt determined that the patients he treated didn't succumb to diseases that plague people in the West. Burkitt hypothesized that the level of fiber intake correlated with risks for cardiovascular diseases, diabetes, varicose veins, constipation, diverticulitis, hemorrhoids, and colorectal cancer. Burkitt's work sparked the interest of scholars from all areas of medical research.

Today, a large catalog of studies details the health benefits of fiber. This super-nutrient has been shown to:

- Lower blood sugar
- Reduce LDL or "bad" cholesterol levels
- Treat constipation
- Manage irritable bowel syndrome
- Prevent and manage diverticulosis
- Boost immune function
- Reduce the incidence of colorectal and breast cancers
- Help with weight loss

Unfortunately, Americans today consume only 50 percent of the fiber needed to maintain good health and to prevent diseases. As I discussed earlier, the carbohydrates we currently eat are largely refined (e.g., white bread and white rice). The American Dietetic Association recommends that men consume between 30 grams and 38 grams of fiber daily and that women aim for between 21 grams and 25 grams per day. Children should eat an amount in grams equal to their age plus 5 grams per day. Table 2-1 lists the fiber contents of common foods.

Table 2-1
Fiber Contents of Common Foods

Food	Amount	Fiber content (grams)
Almonds	½ cup	7
Apple	1 medium	4
Apricots (dried)	½ cup	2
Banana	1 medium	3
Blackberries	½ cup	4
Broccoli (fresh, cooked)	¾ cup	7
Kidney beans (cooked)	1 cup	19
Oatmeal	1 cup	4
Orange	1 large	2
Pear	1 medium	4
Whole wheat bread	1 slice	3
Yam (cooked or baked with skin)	1 medium	6

Healthy Proteins

Protein supplies nutrients needed to repair connective tissues damaged by normal daily activities. Every cell, tissue, organ and bodily fluids contain protein. We should consume about 20 percent of our calories from protein or approximately 0.8 grams of protein per kilogram (2.2 pounds) of body weight. Excessive protein consumption, a fad practiced by some fitness enthusiasts, can stress the kidneys and can potentially lead to kidney disease as well as excessive calcium loss. Aim for healthy forms of protein such as beans, tofu, tempeh, soy milk, fish, turkey, and fat-free dairy products.

Beans. From Edamame to Garbanzo, beans pack a healthy nutrition punch, proving that good things do come in small packages. Extensive research has shown that a diet containing beans effectively lowers the risk for heart disease and some cancers.

The seven most popular beans in the United States are: Garbanzo, Lima, navy, kidney, edamame, pinto and black beans. Garbanzo beans (also called chickpeas) are high in protein, fiber, iron and calcium. Besides protein, lima beans contain potassium, molybdenum, and insoluble fiber.

Navy beans are a good source of thiamine (vitamin B1), iron, calcium and folate. Kidney beans contain vitamin K and iron. Besides omega-3 fatty acids, edamame (green soybean) contains all the essential amino acids—the building blocks of protein. Pinto beans are rich in folate, fiber and antioxidants. Finally, black beans are loaded with heart-healthy antioxidants.

Tofu. Tofu is a popular Japanese food of ancient Chinese origin. It is made by coagulating soy milk before pressing the resulting curd into blocks (similar to the production of cheese from milk). Tofu comes in three forms: silken, soft and firm. One of the original super foods, tofu is packed with nutrients but low in calories. It contains healthy protein, calcium, vitamins, enzymes, and soy isoflavones (which can mimic estrogen). Tofu is quite bland but easy to digest and contains no cholesterol or saturated fat. It's praised for its role in preventing heart disease, osteoporosis, and some cancers.

Tempeh. Tempeh is made via a fermentation process that binds cooked soybeans into a compact cake form. Because tempeh retains whole soybeans, it has a higher protein and fiber content than tofu. Popular around the world, tempeh is delicious and is the leading source of protein for vegans and vegetarians. Like tofu, it provides soy isoflavones and contains no cholesterol or saturated fat and is felt to have a role in the prevention of heart disease, osteoporosis and some cancers.

Soy Milk. This type of milk is an alternative to cow's milk. Soy milk contains low-calorie protein and is high in fiber. Its isoflavones and calcium content have been credited with the prevention of heart disease, osteoporosis and some cancers.

Fish. Most nutritionists recommend eating fish twice a week as a healthier alternative to meats and poultry. Fish is low in saturated fats and provides protein, vitamins, and minerals. In addition, cold-water fish, such as salmon, tuna, and sardines provide healthy omega-3 fats, which have been linked to a low risk for heart disease, stroke and some cancers. Omega-3 fats, especially the docosahexaenoic (DHA) type, have been shown to lower blood levels of C-reactive protein (CRP), which is a biomarker linked to heart disease, some cancers, and immune dysfunction.

However, a cautionary note about fish is in order: More and more, fish are found to harbor dangerous levels of mercury, a neurotoxin that is especially dangerous to young children and pregnant and breastfeeding women! Fish at-risk for high mercury levels include big tuna, shark, king mackerel, and swordfish. Fish low in mercury tend to be wild rather than farm-raised and include wild salmon, herring, catfish, tilapia, shrimp and non-farmed trout.

The FDA and the Environmental Protection Agency recommend that women and young children eat no more than 12 ounces (i.e., two servings) per week of fish low in mercury. Additionally, only 6 ounces of fish that tend to be high in mercury, such as Albacore or "white" tuna, should be consumed per week.

Turkey. Turkey has become a favorite low-fat, low-calorie food. Rich in folic acid, B-vitamins, zinc and potassium, turkey is a popular replacement for meats and even chicken. Made popular by Thanksgiving, turkey's one drawback is its dryness.

Fat-free Dairy Products. Milk and other dairy products provide a number of healthy nutrients. Milk is high in protein, potassium, calcium, vitamins A, D, B2, and B12. Protein is needed to repair tissue destroyed by normal daily activities. Low intake of potassium and calcium are connected to high blood pressure. Vitamins A and D have been credited with lowering the risk for some cancers. Riboflavin or Vitamin B2 helps extract energy from carbohydrates, fats and protein. Vitamin B12 works closely with another B vitamin, folate, to synthesize DNA.

However, there is a downside to some forms of dairy products. Indeed, some health experts believe that eliminating dairy products from the diet is the single most important strategy for improving short- and long-term health. Cow's milk is linked to allergies, eczema, and sinus disease. The American Academy of Pediatrics warns that exposure to cow's milk protein in the first few months of an infant's life might be a significant factor in the development of Type 1 diabetes.

Fruits and Vegetables

One of Doug Larson's famous sayings is: "Life expectancy would grow by leaps and bounds if green vegetables smelled as good as bacon." Both fruits and vegetables have achieved "Super Foods" status for good reasons. They are rich sources of vitamins, minerals and phytonutrients. Most are low in fats and calories and are great sources of fiber. Slowly, we are discovering the litany of phytonutrients such as resveratrol, anthocyanin, and lycopene contained in fruits and vegetables.

Population studies are clear in their findings: people who consume lots of fruits and vegetables are at lower risk of developing heart disease, stroke, high blood pressure, some cancers, diabetes, and other degenerative diseases. In a study (dubbed, the "Chample 3 Study") conducted by Dr. Hedemi Todoriki and colleagues at the University of the Ryukyus in Okinawa, Japan, Americans who consumed traditional Okinawan vegetables for only 4 weeks were able to lower their blood pressure, cholesterol, BMI, and other disease-betraying biomarkers.[2]

Numerous other studies have uncovered the disease-preventing properties of vegetables. For instance, green, leafy vegetables can ward off cancers of the mouth, throat, colon and bladder. Lutein and zeaxanthin contained in dark, green vegetables can prevent the development of cataracts and macular degeneration, a leading cause of blindness among the elderly. Carrots contain beta carotene, which has been shown to prevent heart disease. The cruciferous vegetables, including cabbage, kale, bok choy, and Brussels sprouts contain sulforaphane, which has been credited as an immune booster.

When possible, eat unpeeled, raw or steamed fruits and vegetables to get the benefits of all their nutrients, such as enzymes. Chose from a variety of fresh fruits and vegetables—especially the colorful ones, organically grown. Most authorities recommend that adults consume between 5 and 10 servings of fruits and vegetables each and every day. I recommend that you eat more vegetables than fruits to avoid the sugars in fruits.

Healthy Snacks

Most people snack between breakfast, lunch and dinner. In a recent survey, 95 percent of American adults and children eat at least one snack daily. Unfortunately, most snacks are high in calories, sugar, sodium and fat. Most nutritionists recommend *healthy* snacking as a strategic way to reduce overall caloric intake. The rationale is that if you eat your main meals when you are very hungry you'll over eat.

Healthy snacks maintain healthy blood sugar levels and reduce hunger pangs. Even the most finicky eater can find a variety of healthy snacks. Individuals with diabetes, high blood pressure, heart disease and other chronic diseases can find healthy snacks compatible with their condition. You can get downright creative with your snack foods, such as nuts, yogurt, smoothies, fruits and vegetables, popcorn, and trail mixes.

Nuts. There're a large variety of nuts from which to choose. Nuts are great sources of healthy protein, fiber, minerals, phytonutrients and antioxidants. Most contain healthy fats, like the omeg-3 fats. In 2003, the FDA allowed manufacturers of almonds, hazelnuts, peanuts, pecans, walnuts and pistachios to advertize heart health-promoting claims for their products. The only drawback to nuts is that they are high in calories, so be sure to stick to the recommended intake: one handful at a time!

Yogurt. Like nuts, there are a large variety of yogurts from which to choose. Yogurt provides a nice mix of calcium, potassium, protein, and live-bacteria cultures (i.e., probiotics). Adding berries, nuts and raisins can enhance the taste and nutrition value. Studies show that probiotics improve immune function and gastrointestinal health.

Smoothies. Like yogurt, smoothies offer enough varieties to satisfy every taste. A blend of chilled fruits and juice, smoothies contain calcium, potassium, and protein, depending on ingredients. Try these popular drinks as a healthy way to tide you over between meals.

Fruits and Vegetables. I discussed the health benefits of fruits and vegetables in the previous section of this chapter. These are some of the most versatile grab-n-go foods, offering a long list of vitamins, minerals, phytonutrients, and fiber. From celery sticks to apples, fresh fruits and vegetables are some of the most popular snack foods.

Popcorn. Another popular snack, popcorn (without butter), is a healthy snack low in calories and high in fiber. The smell of freshly popped popcorn permeates a room and teases the senses; it is one of the most recognizable smells around! A standard 3-cup serving of air-popped popcorn contains just 93 calories. Beware of some microwave popcorns which can be high in sodium, trans-fats and calories. You're better off with old-fashion air popped popcorn.

Trail Mixes. When it comes to creative snacks, trail mix is at the top of the list! Its goodies include dried fruit, nuts, seeds, raisins, shredded coconut, pretzels, whole-wheat cereal and chocolate. Lightweight and easy to pack, this internationally-renowned, high-energy snack can tide you over until your next big meal. The nutrient value depends on the contents of the mix, but can include protein, fiber, vitamins and minerals. Keep sweets out of your trail mix!

Water

An estimated 65 to 75 percent of the adult human body is composed of water; children's bodies comprise between 85 and 90 percent water, depending on age. Water serves many crucial functions including: regulating body temperature; lubricating joints; facilitating most biochemical processes (e.g., hormone and neurotransmitter production); and serving as a media for transporting nutrients throughout the body.

Despite its importance to basic physiological function, health and nutrition experts estimate that an astounding 50 percent to 75 percent of Americans are chronically dehydrated! This is unbelievable! There are many ways to ensure that you're getting enough fluids daily. The most popular method is to drink eight 12-ounce glasses daily. Another way is to drink enough to ensure that your urine is clear. Finally, you can drink enough healthy fluids to make you urinate every 3 to 4 hours.

Unfortunately, our water supply leaves a lot to be desired. Most experts recommend that you install a reverse osmosis purification system in your house to make drinking water. If you purchase bottled water avoid leaving them in a hot environment. Environmental scientists now identify plastic bottles as sources of dangerous xenoestrogens—novel, man-made compounds that occupy estrogen receptors in the body because their chemical structures mimic naturally-occurring estrogen. Some health experts link xenoestrogens to hormonal imbalances and to the development of breast and other types of cancers.

Supplements for Most People

As you'll learn in Chapter 3, vitamins, minerals, phytonutrients, enzymes, and accessory nutrients are indispensable to good health and wellness. These micronutrients form the basis of nearly all biochemical processes in the body. The best way to get your daily supply of micronutrients is from whole foods, but the vast majority of Americans don't eat healthy enough to get them exclusively from foods. Another factor is that as the body ages, its ability to absorb and use micronutrients diminishes, requiring supplementation as the best way to strategically support myriad biochemical processes.

DEVELOPING GOOD EATING HABITS

Changing the way you eat will be one of your most difficult lifestyle modifications! After all, the way you eat today has its genesis in infancy and childhood and honed over the years. Therefore, you are not going to fundamentally change how and what you eat as an adult without physically and psychologically shocking your system! But it can be done.

Dietary change is an important component of the treatment and prevention of several medical disorders, including diabetes mellitus, osteoporosis, congestive heart failure, and hypertension. Persons diagnosed with high blood pressure, for example, can better manage and even reverse their condition by consuming a comprehensive mix of minerals, ideally through vegetables. In addition, hypertensives should eat foods low in salt and low in calories, if overweight. A blood pressure-lowering diet can also help your anti-hypertensive medication(s) work better.

Fundamental to any dietary modification is behavior modification. Since eating habits are well-ingrained behaviors that begin during infancy and childhood, changing your eating style requires a change in your attitude about food. For example, thinking of food as indispensable nutrient to fuel your activities might help you to select energy-producing food. Thus, our relationship with food is a necessary part of dietary modification. Other strategies crucial to successfully changing your diet include eating mindfully and skillfully dining out, if you so choose.

Develop a Healthy Relationship with Food

Most people who abuse food do so because of an abnormal relationship with food. Few of us can recall the last time we were hungry! We typically employ cues to drive our eating. Indeed, the majority of our eating activities are cued by stress, anxiety, depression, boredom, TV commercials and other automatic triggers. We should adhere to the old adage: Eat to live; not live to eat!

Before you eat, stop and ask yourself whether or not you are really hungry. If you can honestly answer in the affirmative, go ahead and eat. Conversely, if the answer is "no", put away the food and do something else.

Eat Mindfully

Health experts warn that eating on-the-go is dangerous as it invites a number of health problems such as overeating, under nourishment, weight gain, and gastroesophageal reflux disease (GERD).

Most health authorities now recommend mindful eating to facilitate digestion. You should eat slowing and be completely aware of the entire experience. Chew each bite slowly and take 30 minutes to eat your large meals.

Chewing your food slowly and completely are crucial for good digestion. Firstly, chewing mechanically breaks down large food particles into smaller pieces. In addition, chewing slowly allows saliva to evenly mix with the food. Saliva contains bicarbonate, which can help neutralize stomach acid and minimize GERD.

Healthy Dining Out

Americans are increasingly eating meals away from home. Restaurants have become the primary place for individual and family dining, social events, and business meetings. Eating outside the home is not intrinsically bad but you'll have to judiciously select the amount and type of food you consume. Even persons with nutritionally-based chronic diseases such as diabetes and hypertension can eat out relatively healthy.

The following tips can help you make wise choices when dining-out:

- Call ahead and ask if the chef is willing to prepare your meals for you. Most fine restaurants are eager to prepare healthy meals on request.
- Choose only healthy appetizers such as vegetables and fruits. Conversely, you can eat an appetizer before leaving home. Whatever you do, stay away from high-calorie appetizers such as butter-filled rolls.
- For your entree, avoid sauces and gravies. Alternatively, request that sauces be served on the side, giving you the option of serving yourself a small amount.
- Forgo dessert altogether. If you must eat dessert, choose a small portion size from the most healthy available, such as fruit and yogurt.

FOODS AS MEDICINE

Emerging scientific evidence points to food as medicine. These foods are the ones that typically line the periphery of the supermarket and sold as whole foods. Let's now look at: the Okinawa diet; the Mediterranean diet; foods that lower cholesterol; foods that reduce inflammation; and foods that can prevent some types of cancers.

The Okinawa Diet

I live on the Japanese island of Okinawa, which is famous for having the highest concentration of centenarians and super-centenarians on the planet! Older Okinawans adhere to a low-calorie, low-fat, nutrient dense diet with a favorable omega-3 to omega-6 ratio. In fact, this way of eating is widely credited with contributing to the exceptional longevity observed among Okinawa's elderly population.

Low in unhealthy fats and meats, the traditional Okinawan way of eating is high in fish, green and yellow vegetables, grains, soybean and other legumes, and sweet potatoes. This high-fiber diet imparts a healthy mix of minerals, vitamins and phytonutrients. The bestselling book, *The Okinawa Diet Plan*, is a comprehensive eating plan that offers 160 recipes for dishes that promote health and prevent lifestyle diseases such as high blood pressure, diabetes, osteoarthritis, and some cancers. See Appendix II for more information on buying this splendid book.

The Mediterranean Diet

The so-called Mediterranean Diet is characterized by a high intake of complex carbohydrates (e.g., fiber), low-calorie protein, mono-unsaturated fats, vitamins, minerals, and phytonutrients. This style of eating emphasizes a high intake of fruits, vegetables, cereals, potatoes, fish, poultry, beans, nuts, and olive oil. Drawn from the dietary habits of people living in and around the Mediterranean, this approach to eating de-emphasizes the intake of red meat, milk, and saturated fats.

Foods That Lower Cholesterol

Most people know that foods that contain saturated and trans-fats can raise cholesterol levels. However, few people are aware that eating the right foods can actually lower cholesterol.

Garlic. This original super herb has been celebrated for centuries for its wide-ranging medicinal properties. In ancient times, garlic was cherished for its ability to enhance strength and endurance. Today, the organosulfur compounds in garlic that give it its pungent odor are recognized for their health promoting and disease fighting eclecticism.

For example, a study published in 1995 in the *British Journal of Clinical Research* showed that garlic effectively reduced cholesterol and blood pressure in test subjects.[3]

Fiber. As discussed earlier in this chapter, one of the numerous health benefits of dietary fiber is its ability to reduce total and LDL cholesterol levels.

Flaxseed. This "Super Food" is high in fiber and contains alpha linoleic acid, an Omega-3 essential fatty acid that has been shown to increase levels of HDL cholesterol and lower LDL cholesterol.

Olive Oil. Studies have shown that 2 to 3 tablespoons of virgin olive oil per day can decrease LDL cholesterol.

Soy. Numerous scientific studies show that these products, which include tofu, tempeh and soy milk, can lower LDL cholesterol.[4]

Foods that Reduce Inflammation

Scientists and clinicians now agree that inflammation is the basis for a long list of chronic diseases such as heart disease, stroke, and cancer. An important strategy in combating these inflammatory conditions is adhering to an anti-inflammatory diet. The following is generally accepted as the elements of an anti-inflammatory diet:

- Eat a variety of foods from all macronutrients and micronutrients food groups.
- Aim for organic foods as much as possible.
- Eliminate processed foods.
- Eliminate trans-fats.
- Avoid foods with high fructose corn syrup.

- Minimize dairy products.
- Adhere to your daily calorie requirement. A rough way to calculate your caloric requirement is to multiply your ideal body weight (IBW) by 13, 14 or 15, depending on your level of activity. If you are sedentary multiply your IBW by 13; if you exercise most days of the week, multiply your IBW by 14; use 15 if you engage in high-level physical fitness programs.
- Eat 10 servings of fruits and vegetables, daily.
- Aim for the following distribution of macronutrients: 40 to 50 percent of calories from complex carbohydrates; 30 percent from healthy fats; and 20 to 30 percent from healthy proteins.
- For carbohydrates, aim for more whole grains, beans, and sweet potatoes.
- For protein, stick to fish, turkey, chicken, and soy products.
- For fats, use foods with omega-3 fatty acids such as olive, canola, and grape seed oils.
- Take a pharmaceutical grade multivitamin/multimineral supplement daily.

Foods that Prevent Cancer

A rapidly emerging area of nutrition science is our understanding of how foods help prevent the development of some types of cancers by protecting our DNA and activate certain genes. These foods contain phytochemicals, a group of over 10,000 plant-derived nutrients that have been shown to promote health and prevent disease.

Saponins. These are a group of naturally occurring, complex compounds found in plants, particularly desert plants such as *Yucca schidigera* and

Quillaja saponaria. Saponins work to help a plant's immune system ward off microbial agents. Recent research in humans shows that saponins enhance immune function and beat back some types of cancer cells. Additionally, saponins show antimicrobial activities against fungi, protozoa, viruses, and bacteria. Foods high in saponins include soybeans, peas, oats, and alfalfa sprouts.

Anthocyanins. These are a large group of more than 500 known complex compounds found in plants, fruits and flowers, especially berries and grapes. Anthocyanins give plants, fruits, and flowers their brilliant pigment which protects against severe conditions such as hot sun, heavy wind, and torrential rain. Emerging research in human subjects suggests that anthocyanins have anti-inflammatory, antioxidant, antimicrobial and anti-cancer properties.[5] Foods high in anthocyanins include blueberries, blackberries, black grapes, beets, dark cherries, purple carrots, purple sweet potatoes, pomegranate, and acai fruit.

Carotenoids. The carotenoids are a group of over 600 fat-soluble compounds found mostly in plants and algae, and serving primarily to absorb light energy for photosynthesis and to protect chlorophyll from damage by light and oxygen. The carotenoids are categorized into xanthophylls and carotenes. In humans, beta carotene acts as a precursor to vitamin A, an important nutrient for night vision and a super antioxidant. Carotenoids also appear to facilitate communication between cells.

The antioxidant property of carotenoids protects DNA against mutation and cancer.[6] In one study, however, beta carotene supplement was linked to an increased risk for lung cancer in smokers.[7] Lycopene has been credited with reducing the risk for prostate and breast cancer. Foods high in carotenoids include tomatoes, carrots, sweet potatoes, collard greens, spinach, and kale.

Fiber. As discussed earlier in this chapter, one of the numerous health benefits of dietary fiber is its ability to reduce the risk of colorectal and breast cancers. I recommend that you review this section, if needed.

Mushrooms. Mushrooms are one of the oldest health foods, with a lineage that dates back over 1,000 years. Credited by the ancient Greek for providing strength in battle, the Romans regarded mushrooms and a gift from God. The Chinese embraced mushrooms (and still do today) for their medicinal properties.

Of the nearly 14,000 types of mushrooms, only 3,000 are considered edible. Commonly classified as a vegetable and an herb, mushrooms, technically speaking, are fungi. It is flexible enough to be used in soups, salads, casseroles or as an appetizer. Low in sodium, fat and calories, mushrooms are rich in vitamins, minerals and contain phytochemicals, such as the strong antioxidants ergothionene, and polyphenols.

Dietary mushrooms have been linked to a reduced risk for breast and prostate cancers.[8] Mushrooms likely reduce cancer risk via their antioxidant properties. In addition, beta-glucans, a type of soluble fiber found in mushrooms, is felt to boost immune function.

Super Fruit Juices

In the past two decades or so, a number of fruit juices have emerged on the American market, mostly via network marketing. These juices contain phytochemicals, powerful antioxidants that mitigate the damage of free radicals, boost energy, prevent heart disease, and help fight cancer and other diseases. ExFuze, a relatively new company, has smartly blended the juices from multiple super fruits and berries to create Seven-plus: acai berry, goji berry, mangos teen fruit, noni fruit, seabuckthorn berry, and gac fruit. Let's now take a look at each one of these super fruits/berries:

Acai Berry Juice. One of the most studied of the super juices is acai juice derived from the acai berry. This berry packs an impressive array of phytonutrients that are increasingly being credited with promoting health and preventing disease. It contains catechins (similar to levels found in green tea); anthocyanins (10 to 30 times more anthocyanins that red wine); essential fatty acids (similar to levels found in olive oil); and Phytosterols. Acai berry also contains amino acids; vitamins A, B, C, and E; and fiber. Additionally, this berry has a low glycemic index.

The nutrients in acai berry do a body good! Bestselling author and anti-aging physician, Dr. Nicholas Perricone, remarked in his book *The Perricone Promise* that acai juice is the #1 super food of his list of super foods! I agree with Dr. Perricone—this berry, found in the Amazon rainforest, is remarkably nutritious!

Goji Berry Juice. This super juice has been featured in numerous newspapers and on many television shows, including CNN, ABC, and on the Oprah Show. It attained super food status because it contains a long list of health promoting and disease preventing phytonutrients. Found mostly in the Himalayas, this berry was credited with helping ancient Chinese live a long time.

The Goji berry (also called Wolfberry) is rich in amino acids, carotenoids, minerals, vitamins, zeaxanthin and essential fatty acids. These nutrients have been shown to lower LDL cholesterol (the so-called "bad" cholesterol), improve cognitive function, and slow the aging process. Preliminary laboratory studies that this berry might have activities against cancer cells. Goji juice can thin the blood so people taking blood thinners (e.g., warfarin) should avoid Goji berries and juice. Goji berry may interact negatively with diabetes and high blood pressure medications.

Mangosteen Fruit Juice. This fruit, found naturally in Southeast Asia, contains 43 different Xanthones and is loaded with antioxidants. Popular in Asian countries for hundreds of years, Mangosteen is believed to help digestion, fight allergies, reduce inflammation and strengthen the immune system.

Noni Fruit Juice. This fruit, native to the South Pacific islands, contains an impressive array of phytonutrients, such as vitamins A, B, C and D, minerals and amino acids. Numerous studies have credited juice from this fruit with helping to manage bronchitis, arthritis and gum disease. As an antioxidant, Noni can scavenge free radicals and create a healthy environment in the body. Popular as an energy booster, Noni juice is believed to impart antiviral, antifungal, antibacterial, and antitumor benefits.

Seabuckthorn Berry Juice. Found in both Asia and Europe, the Seabuckthorn berry is rich in vitamins, minerals, and essential fatty acids. It's commonly used to treat skin and digestive disorders. Seabuckthorn has anti-inflammatory, antimicrobial, and analgesic activities and promotes tissue regeneration. Seabuckthorn oil is used to treat eczema and burns.

Gac Fruit Juice. This fruit is popular in Vietnam where it is served on special occasions. It has an impressive phytonutritional profile and is known for its high levels of lycopene. In fact, the Gac fruit has 70 times more lycopene than tomato or watermelon. Additionally, this super fruit contains 10 times the beta-carotene of sweet potatoes or carrots. In Vietnam, the seed membranes of the gac fruit are used to treat dry eyes. Its antioxidants reportedly have skin healing properties that rejuvenate lackluster skin.

HOW TO LOSE FIVE POUNDS IN THE NEXT 30 DAYS

In the past two decades or so it has become painfully clear that diets don't work. As Dr. Andrew Weil is fond of saying "diets are things that you eventually stop." When you stop even the most successful diet, you revert back to your normal style of eating and quickly return to your previous weight. The best way to ensure sustained and permanent weight loss is to develop the daily habit of a healthy lifestyle. The following represents a synthesis of healthy ways of living based on current scientific evidence:

- Eat breakfast. After fasting all night, the last thing you want to do is to keep fasting. Skipping breakfast has been shown to slow your metabolism and body's fat-burning capacity. Choose from a variety of food groups.

- Eat two healthy snacks at 10:00 am and 2:00 pm. This strategy can help rev up your metabolism and reduce the tendency to overeat. As discussed earlier, healthy snack choices include a variety of nuts, yogurt, smoothies, fruits and vegetables, popcorn, and trail mixes.

- Eat 10 servings of vegetables and fruits each day. Vegetables and fruits offer unique phytonutrients that support health and wellness. Many of these micronutrients are still being discovered and their roles are yet to be defined.

- Drink enough water to urinate every 3 to 4 hours or so. Water forms the basic biochemical environment for optimal physiological reactions in the body.

- Consume 200 calories less from each dinner. This helps you shave off calories from your total intake at the most strategic time of the day (i.e., when you are least active).

- 3 days each week: NO sweets, cakes, pastries, breads. This reduces your weekly burden of simple carbohydrates, a move that can help lower your insulin resistance profile.

- Take a multivitamin/multimineral supplement daily. As I'll discuss in the next chapter, this strategy can help fill gaps in your nutrition and lays the foundation for healthy aging by augmenting cell function.

- Sleep 7 to 9 hours each night. Adequate quality and quantity of sleep has global health and wellness benefits and help your body achieve and maintain a healthy weight (see Chapter 6).

- Review your list of "blessings" at start of each day. This can help mitigate your stress levels, boost self-esteem and prevent over eating. (see Chapter 7).
- Spend 5 minutes of quiet, "me" time every 4 hours. A few minutes of periodic respite has been show to break the cycle of stress that invariably characterizes our day.
- Accumulate at least 10,000 steps on a step counter/pedometer each day. This translates to about three miles of physical activity daily (see Chapter 4).
- As bestselling author, Michael Pollan advices, "Eat food, not too much, mostly plants."

IN SUMMARY

- Nutrition is a major underlying principle of good health, wellness, and longevity as well as a long list of chronic diseases.
- A wellness-centric and longevity-supporting nutrition practices are:
    - Three balanced meals and three or four healthy snacks each day
    - Five to 10 servings of vegetables and fruits daily.
    - Minimize intake of saturated and the so-called trans-fats.
    - Eat only low-calorie protein from fish, beans, and tofu; complex carbohydrates.
    - Minimize sodium and sugar intake

    - Get adequate amounts of calcium, magnesium, and potassium, preferably from whole foods
    - Avoid dining out, if possible.

- You can develop healthy nutrition practices by: developing a good relationship with food; mindful eating and skillfully eating out.
- Food is medicine, and traditional eating styles such as those of the elderly of Okinawa and the Mediterranean can lower blood pressure, blood lipids, and inflammation and prevent certain cancers.
- You can potentially drop significant amounts of weight by: eating breakfast lunch and dinner; two healthy snacks; 10 servings of vegetables and fruits; drinking enough water; omitting 200 calories from dinner and sweets three days a week; and taking a daily multivitamin/mineral supplement. Additionally, you can lose weight via: reviewing a list of your blessings each day; spending 5 minutes of "me" time every 4 hours; and accumulating 10,000 steps daily.

Chapter 3

Take Selected Dietary Supplements

"In the recent past, medical authorities told consumers that supplements were a waste of money. Now they say they are dangerous, even life threatening, foisted on a gullible public by an unregulated industry that cares only about profit and is heedless of the harm it causes. On the other side are health experts, including some physicians, who recommend dietary supplements enthusiastically. Some of them are brilliant scientists."
—Dr. Andrew Weil
New York Times bestselling author of eleven books, including *Healthy Aging*

One of the most contentious areas of health and wellness in the past two decades has been the routine use of dietary supplements by the general population. Conflicting scientific studies abound. Some research shows that nutritional supplements optimize health and prevent disease while others show no benefits or even harm. This leaves the public wondering if the average North American should take a daily dietary supplement or avoid them altogether. Are vitamins and minerals important for health and wellness? Are supplements a waste of money? Are they harmful? These questions have engaged scientists, clinicians, health educators, policy makers, and others in lively debate.

The American Dietetic Association (ADA) recommends that food should always be a person's primary source of micronutrients such as vitamins, minerals, and *phytonutrients*. Medical and nutrition experts unanimously agree with the ADA, as do I. However, the reality is that few Americans eat in a manner that would provide them with the needed micronutrients and phytonutrients exclusively from their diet. A national survey sponsored by the National Center for Health Statistics found that only 30 percent of Americans consume the requisite servings of fruits and vegetables needed to get the recommended daily value (DV) of vitamins, minerals, and phytonutrients.[1] Most authorities agree that our soil is woefully depleted of the minerals (e.g., selenium) needed to sustain optimum health and wellness. Moreover, much of the foods we consume today are highly processed, which removes fiber, enzymes, vitamins, and minerals. Finally, the toxic environment in which many of us live demands additional micronutrient protection, especially from *antioxidants*. Therefore, most Americans have gaps in their day-to-day nutritional status.

These troubling trends prompted two prominent researchers from Harvard University to recommend in an article published in June 2002 in the *Journal of the American Medical Association* that most adult Americans should take a multivitamin daily. World-renowned integrative medicine expert, Dr. Andrew Weil, director of the Integrative Medicine Program at the University of Arizona, recommends that most Americans supplement their diet with selected vitamins, minerals and accessory nutrients.[2] Other prominent experts, who share Dr. Weil's opinion, include: Dr. Julian Whitaker of the Whitaker Wellness Institute in Newport Beach, California; Dr. Steven Hotze of the Hotze Health & Wellness Center in Houston, Texas; Dr. Michael Lam, director of education at the Academy of Anti-Aging Research; and Dr. Elson Haas of the Preventive Medicine Center in Marin, California.

Again, it should be made crystal clear that the cornerstone of good nutrition is a balanced diet that includes five to ten servings of fruits and vegetables, fiber, and healthy macronutrients; not dietary supplements. Indeed, taking supplements in the face of poor eating habits will not accrue good health. I believe that taking nutritional supplements should be regarded as an insurance policy to fill gaps in our nutritional status—which is the case for 70 percent of Americans.

Additionally, as I'll delineate in this chapter, very good medical research is beginning to show that vitamins, minerals, and other supplements effectively prevent, mitigate, or manage certain diseases—including osteoporosis, heart disease, neurological diseases, and some cancers.

WHAT ARE DIETARY SUPPLEMENTS?

Dietary supplements have been sold in the United States for many decades in pill, powder, and liquid forms, but their use has recently become a health lightening rod. Just what are these nutrients that have become the source of so much controversy of late? Firstly, let me reaffirm that vitamins and minerals are absolutely crucial to the workings of every functional cell in the human body! In fact, the word vitamin is derived from the words *vital* and *amine* because scientists who first discovered these micronutrients realized how vital they were to health and life. (As it turned out, not all vitamins are amines but the suffix amine remains to this day).

The internationally-acclaimed Linus Pauling Institute at the University of Oregon declares that every cell in the human body requires vitamins and minerals each and every day to drive the myriad biochemical functions. Some vitamins and minerals serve as *antioxidants* to help protect enzymes, cell membranes and DNA from damage by *free radicals*, which are toxic by-products produced in the body during metabolism. Others serve as templates for normal growth and development. For example, folic acid, a water-soluble B-vitamin, effectively lowers the risk of severe birth defects such as spina bifida in newborns—a major public health problem. Vitamin D/calcium combination reduces the risk of fractures in people with *osteoporosis* or thinning of the bones.

In the 1940s, the U.S. Food and Nutrition Board established the well-known recommended daily allowance (now referred to as the daily value or DV), the minimum amount of vitamins and minerals needed to prevent disease. Adopted by the U.S. Food and Drug Administration, the DV has become the standard recommendation for daily nutrient intake for a healthy person (Tables 3-1 and 3-2). Many prominent nutritionists, however, recommend additional amounts of these micronutrients for people with certain health conditions, based on emerging scientific and anecdotal evidence that vitamins, minerals, and other nutritional supplements can mitigate or prevent a long list of diseases and conditions. For instance, the DV for vitamin C is 75 mg for women and 90 mg for men daily, but experts recommend 200 mg per day to facilitate optimal health and wellness.

Supplements come in doses of micrograms (1 millionth of a gram), milligram (1 thousandth of a gram) or grams. The fat-soluble vitamins (i.e., vitamins A, D, E, and K) usually come in International Units or IU (1 IU is about 1 milligram).

Vitamins

There are thirteen known vitamins: A, B-complex (made up of 8 vitamins), C, D, E, and K. Found mostly in fruits and vegetables, vitamins are organic compounds that serve as co-factors in myriad biochemical processes. These processes include: energy production; repair and maintenance of cartilage and other tissue; synthesis of genetic materials (i.e., RNA and DNA); and the regulation of blood sugar, thyroid hormones, and other metabolic functions. For example, vitamin B1 (thiamine) and vitamin B3 (niacin) help extract energy from carbohydrates, fats and protein. Without these vitamins, you'd feel chronically fatigued and be weakened from lack of energy and vitality—regardless of how well you eat.

Minerals

Minerals are inorganic substances (e.g., metals) that are necessary for health and life. These nutrients originate in the earth and can't be manufactured by the body. We obtain most of our minerals from plant-based foods and some from animals-based foods. Like vitamins, minerals serve as co-factors in myriad biochemical processes. These processes include: the repair and maintenance of bones and other tissue; the maintenance of nerve function; energy production; and the regulation of blood sugar, thyroid hormones, and other metabolic processes. Chromium, for example, helps regulate blood sugar while potassium and magnesium help with nerve function. Without these minerals, you'd feel chronically sluggish and develop neurological symptoms such as tingling and numbness.

Accessory Nutrients

Accessory nutrients are a diverse group of nutrients that have central roles in health maintenance and life extension, similar to vitamins and minerals. They are dubbed "accessory" because they are neither vitamins nor minerals and there is no single category established for them. Accessory nutrients include amino acids, co-enzymes, and plant pigments. Co-enzyme Q-10, one of the most studied nutritional supplements, is an indispensable co-factor in energy production. L-Carnitine is an amino acid that is also crucial to energy production. The omega-3 fatty acids are probably the most written about and talked about nutritional supplements in the past decade due to the growing list of impressive benefits credited to these so-called healthy fats. Indeed, accessory nutrients are rapidly emerging as the mainstay of human health and wellness.

VITAMINS FROM A TO Z

As I discussed earlier, vitamins are indispensable to health and life; without them you'll develop disease and die. Vitamins can be characterized as fat-soluble or water-soluble. The fat-soluble vitamins are A, D, E and K. The eight B vitamins, as well as vitamin C, are water-soluble. Fat-soluble vitamins absorb better into the body with help of a little fat in the meal, and should therefore be taken after a high-fat meal. Water-soluble vitamins have no such requirement.

Since multivitamins typically combine both fat-soluble and water-soluble vitamins, I recommend you take your multivitamins after a high-fat meal. It should be noted that the body can store fat-soluble vitamins for months, which can potentially rise to toxic levels. So, please check with your healthcare provider before you exceed the RDA of fat-soluble vitamins. On the other hand, excess amounts of water-soluble vitamins are excreted in the urine (assuming your kidneys are working properly) and there's very little danger in them accumulating to toxic levels.

Vitamin A

Vitamin A is a fat-soluble vitamin with a long list of important biological functions. It is present in the body in various forms including retinol, retinal, and the carotenoids (such as beta-carotene, lycopene and lutein). Best known for its role in maintaining night vision and preventing macular degeneration (deterioration of the central part of the retina that leads to blindness), this vitamin also has roles in boosting the immune system, building strong bones and teeth, and keeping the skin healthy. Vitamin A also has clinical, disease-fighting applications, most notably its role in treating skin disorders such as acne, psoriasis, eczema, and burns.

This antioxidant vitamin may also help minimize the acute effects of an upper respiratory infection, alleviate dry eyes, promote thyroid function, and supplement the management of chronic lung disease. The *carotenoids,* a group of compounds that are precursors of vitamin A, are gaining popularity for their impressive health benefits. One of the most well-known carotenoids, lycopene, has been shown to have a role in preventing breast and prostate cancers. Another popular carotenoid is beta carotene which has been shown to boost immune function. Results of a study published in the January 2006 issue of the *American Journal of Clinical Nutrition* indicate that carotenoid supplementation provides protection against DNA damage.[3]

A deficiency in this nutrient manifests as night blindness, brittle hair, and dry skin. Vitamin A can be found abundantly in green, red, orange and yellow fruits and vegetables, animal liver, fish liver oils, egg yolk, and fortified milk. Vitamin A-rich herbs include kelp, chickweed, sage, and yellow dock. The DV for vitamin A is 2,300 IU for adult women and 3,000 IU for adult men but the optimal dose for people with skin conditions such as psoriasis is 5,000-10,000 IU daily.

Pregnant women, the elderly, and people with liver disease should not consume more than 5,000 IU per day. Doses over 50,000 IU per day can result in toxicity, which manifests as headaches, hair loss, joint pain, and gastrointestinal distress. Toxic doses of vitamin A during pregnancy have been implicated in birth defects such as cleft palate and heart defects.

Vitamin B Complex

Why is vitamin B so complex? Well, it really isn't complex, but is actually eight water-soluble vitamins in one that are involved in complex biochemical functions in the body. From counteracting the effects of stress to helping with energy metabolism and the production of hormones, this family of vitamins is as indispensable as any other vitamin. Vitamin B complex is made up of thiamin (B1), riboflavin (B2), niacin (B3), pantothenic acid (B5), pyridoxine (B6), cyanocobalamin (B12), folic acid and biotin.

Although the B vitamins are present in many foods (e.g., eggs, fish, meats, and whole grains), some experts believe that vitamin B deficiency is more common than is generally assumed. Microwave cooking can destroy some B vitamins. A long list of drugs such as estrogens, anti-inflammatory agents, antacids, antibiotics, anti-diabetics, and anti-high blood pressure medicines can deplete some vitamin B levels. Many people over the age of 60 have decreased stomach acid and reduced production of "good" bacteria that help extract vitamin B12 from foods.

Let's take a closer look at the roles of each member of the vitamin B family.

Vitamin B1 (Thiamin or Thiamine). This vitamin is involved in many complex processes such as converting the carbohydrates in foods into energy and production of hydrochloric acid which helps in digestion of foods. Thiamin also helps maintain healthy nerves and muscles, and promotes cognitive function.

Thiamine deficiency is characterized by irritability, depression, fatigue, forgetfulness, loss of appetite, nausea, tingling, and muscle weakness. Excess alcohol consumption blocks the absorption of thiamin. Vitamin B1 is found in a variety of plant and animal foods including nuts, legumes, brown rice, egg yolk, liver, pork, oysters, and dried brewer's yeast. Other sources are broccoli, kelp, spinach, parsley, sage, and asparagus. The DV for this nutrient for adults is 1.5 mg but the optimal dose is 50-100 mg daily.

Vitamin B2 (Riboflavin). Identified in 1933, riboflavin helps extract energy from carbohydrates, fats and protein. In addition, it helps the body synthesize thyroid hormone, helps with the production of red blood cells, and helps with tissue maintenance and repair. Clinically, vitamin B2 is used with vitamin B6 to help manage carpal tunnel syndrome.

Riboflavin deficiency is manifested as redness of the eyes; sores at the corners of the mouth; burning of the lips and tongue; skin rash; hair loss; and insomnia. Common food sources of vitamin B2 are legumes, fish, meat, poultry, milk, spinach, and whole grains. The DV for this nutrient for adults is 15 mg but the optimal dose is 50 mg daily.

Vitamin B3 (Niacin, Niacinamide, Nicotinic Acid). Niacin gained acclaim as a cholesterol-lowering agent but it is involved in dozens of diverse biochemical processes including energy production and hormone synthesis. Many clinicians prescribe this water-soluble vitamin to increase HDL (so-called "good") cholesterol and lower LDL (so-called "bad") cholesterol and triglycerides. There is some preliminary evidence that niacin can reduce the effects of depression, arthritis, and other diseases.

Dietary sources of niacin include red meat, fish, turkey, chicken, eggs, soybeans, broccoli, carrots, and grains. The DV for this nutrient is 14 mg for women and 16 mg for men but up to 1,000 mg daily may be need for specific problems such as high total cholesterol and low HDL cholesterol. Niacin supplements higher than 250 mg per dose may cause a flushed feeling in some individuals. You can minimize niacin-induced hot flushes by drinking plenty of water, eating a handful of nuts, or taking a low-dose aspirin with the supplement. However, before taking aspirin, consult your healthcare provider. Another strategy is to avoid spicy foods and alcohol.

You should consult your healthcare provider before taking niacin if you have glaucoma, low blood pressure, diabetes, liver disease, gout, bleeding disorders, or ulcers. If you are prescribed high doses of niacin for an extended period of time, you should have your liver enzymes measured a few weeks after you start taking the vitamin and every three months or so thereafter.

Vitamin B5 (Pantothenic Acid). The name pantothenic acid is derived from the Greek root *pantos* meaning "everywhere." Indeed, vitamin B5 is found in many plant and animal products. Pantothenic acid works with biotin to release energy from carbohydrates, fats, and proteins and helps the body to synthesize a number of enzymes, hormones and neurotransmitters. Preliminary evidence points to its possible role in helping to manage the symptoms of migraine headaches, stress, heartburn, and chronic fatigue syndrome.

Pantothenic acid deficiency results in fatigue, skin rash, lack of coordination, staggering gait, and restlessness. Vitamin B5 is found in fish, poultry, yogurt, brewer's yeast, legumes, and whole grains. There is no DV for this nutrient but experts recommend between 100 mg and 500 mg daily to help manage specific conditions, such as migraines and stress.

Vitamin B6 (Pyridoxine). This eclectic vitamin is a catalyst in myriad biological processes in the body such as the manufacture of *serotonin* (a substance that helps transmit information between brain cells), red blood cells, proteins and protein-based compounds such as hormones and enzymes. Doctors prescribe vitamin B6 to treat a number of ailments, including premenstrual syndrome (PMS), carpal tunnel syndrome, and asthma.

Because birth control pills deplete pyridoxine in some people, women who take contraceptive pills should ensure adequate intake of this vitamin. Other medications that can deplete vitamin B6 include: the anti-tuberculosis drugs, isoniazid and cycloserine; the anti-Parkinson drug, L-dopa; and the metal chelator, penicillamine. Strict vegetarians might be at risk for vitamin B6 deficiency. Pyridoxine deficiency produces insomnia, lethargy, anxiety, depression and numbness and tingling in the distribution of nerves.

Food sources of vitamin B6 include baked potato, turkey, chicken, organ meats, hazelnuts, and fortified cereals. The DV for this nutrient is 1.3 mg for men and women younger than age 50; 1.5 mg for women over 50; and 1.7 mg for men over 50. The optimal vitamin B6 dose is 50 mg to 100 mg daily for conditions like PMS, morning sickness, depression, and carpal tunnel syndrome. Toxicity, characterized by tingling in the hands and feet, can occur with doses over 200 mg per day.

Vitamin B12 (Cyanocobalamin). This water-soluble vitamin works closely with another B vitamin, folate, to synthesize DNA, form blood cells, and to maintain the myelin sheath (i.e., the protective covering) that surrounds nerve cells. It also helps to convert food into energy, and to strengthen the immune system.

The absorption of cyanocobalamin requires adequate amounts of stomach acid and intrinsic factor (found in the stomach), both of which are depleted as you age. Therefore, older adults should take a vitamin B12 supplement daily. Strict vegetarians (vegans) are at risk for vitamin B12 deficiency and should also supplement their diet with cyanocobalamin. Diabetics and people with multiple sclerosis should also supplement their diet with this vitamin to help protect their nerves from damage. People who suffer from acne rosacea might also benefit from vitamin B12 supplementation.

Deficiency of cyanocobalamin manifests as anemia, dizziness, difficulty maintaining one's balance, numbness or tingling in the arms or legs, confusion, agitation, hallucinations, and dementia. Sources of the vitamin include fish, meat, poultry, milk, cheese, and eggs. The DV for this nutrient is 2.4 μg for all adults but the optimal dose for specific problems, such as the protection of nerves in diabetics, is between 400 μg and 1000 μg daily. There are no known toxic effects of vitamin B12, even when taken in amounts several times the DV.

Biotin. This member of the B-complex group of vitamins, previously named vitamin B7, is synthesized by bacteria in the large intestines. Biotin is an important player in the regulation of blood sugar and the metabolism of carbohydrates, fats, and proteins. Other roles of this B vitamin include promoting healthy sweat glands and bone marrow. Biotin works in concert with Pantothenic acid, folic acid, and vitamin B12 in the production of energy.

Biotin deficiency manifests as hair loss and a red, scaly rash around the eyes, nose, eyes, and genitals. Natural sources of biotin include whole grains, meats, milk, poultry, saltwater fish, and soybeans. There is no DV for biotin but an adequate daily intake is between 35 μg and 60 μg. There are no known toxic effects of biotin.

Folic Acid. This water soluble B vitamin (also called folate) is needed to make and repair RNA and DNA, the building blocks of human cells. Humans also need folate to make red blood cells and to moderate the level of homocysteine in the blood. First identified in the 1930s, this vitamin has become a superstar among nutrition supplements. Its role in preventing severe birth defect of the brain and spinal cord is firmly established.[4]

Thanks to the efforts of public health experts such as Dr. Godfrey Oakley, MD, professor of epidemiology at Emory University's Rollins School of Public Health, enrichment of breads, cereals and other foods with folate has resulted in a 30 percent reduction in incidence of spina bifida among newborns in the past 20 years. It is now standard prenatal practice for healthcare providers to prescribe folate to all pregnant patients. Women who fail to get at least 600 μg of folic acid during the early weeks of pregnancy run a high risk of giving birth to a baby with spina bifida and anencephaly. In fact, women with childbearing plans should start taking folate *before* they become pregnant.

Folate's health benefits don't end with pregnancy and newborn health. In the Nurses' Health Study, women who consumed high amounts of folic acid effectively cut their risk for colon cancer by an impressive 75 percent.[5] In another study published in the October 2005 issue of the *American Journal of Clinical Nutrition*, 800 μg of folic acid reduced blood homocysteine levels by an impressive 23 percent.[6] As you probably know, homocysteine is now regarded as a blood marker for heart disease, stroke, and inflammation. Still, other studies hint that folic acid may protect women who drink excessive alcohol against the development of breast cancer. Finally, a study in the Netherlands concluded that adults who consumed folic acid supplements suffered less hearing loss than those taking a placebo.

Folic acid deficiency leads to anemia, loss of appetite, weight loss, sore tongue, headaches, irritability, and heart palpitations. Folate is found naturally in leafy green vegetables (e.g., spinach, asparagus, and turnip greens), citrus fruits, and dried beans and peas. Breakfast cereals, breads, flours and other grain products are now certified with folic acid. Children, adolescents and adults should consume at least 400 μg of folic acid per day and pregnant women need 600 μg daily.

Vitamin C

Vitamin C (ascorbic acid), a water-soluble vitamin, is the major antioxidant in the body. It scavenges *free radicals*, which are negatively charged molecules that have been linked to cellular dysfunction, believed to be the basis for chronic diseases such as stroke, heart disease, and some cancers. Vitamin C also raises levels of glutathione, an important antioxidant produced by the body. Vitamin C also promotes wound healing and strengthens ligaments, tendons, cartilage and gums.

By protecting the airway from damage by free radicals, vitamin C may help improve the management of asthma. Researchers at the Asthma and Allergy Research Institute in Nedlands, Western Australia report a significant correlation between severe asthma and levels of vitamin C intake. Hay fever, which shares some immunological features of asthma, can be attenuated by high intake of vitamin C.[7] Its antihistamine-like properties make vitamin C a favorite in helping reduce the severity and duration of the common cold.

High ascorbic acid levels in the blood apparently help control blood pressure. Researchers at Boston University School of Medicine and the Linus Pauling Institute at Oregon State University reported a positive correlation between adequate intake of vitamin C and a drop in blood pressure. No one is sure about the mechanism of action, but it might have to do with vitamin C's regulation of nitric oxide, a gas that helps dilate blood vessels, which results in the lower pressure of circulating blood.[8]

Ascorbic acid deficiency manifests as bleeding gums, loosened teeth, poor wound healing, general weakness, lethargy and, in chronic cases, scurvy. Vitamin C is a very safe product, obtained mainly from citrus fruits, broccoli, green peppers, tomatoes and dark green vegetables. Supplementation with very large doses—over 2,000 mg a day—can cause abdominal cramps, diarrhea and bloating in some people. This effect is easily remedied by reducing the dose of the vitamin. Exercise caution when taking high-doses of vitamin C with antidiabetic drugs as vitamin C can enhance the actions of these agents.

The DV for vitamin C is 90 mg for men and 75 mg for women but the optimal dose is around 200 mg daily. Dosage up to 2,000 mg per day is needed to treat asthma, hay fever and other specific conditions.

Vitamin D

Vitamin D is a fat-soluble nutrient that exists in several forms (the major ones are vitamin D2 or ergocalciferol and vitamin D3 or cholecalciferol). It has been the subject of numerous essays and editorials in the scientific and lay literature in the past two decades. With an upsurge in incidence of osteoporosis (thinning of the bones), vitamin D, a major player in the formation of bone, has emerged as a public health savior. This vitamin helps regulate the blood levels of calcium and phosphorous, essential elements in the building of strong bones and healthy teeth. Vitamin D has also been credited with helping to augment the immune system, slow the progression of arthritis, and prevent cancers of the breast, prostate, and colon. Australian researchers found that vitamin D supplementation successfully mitigated depressive symptoms among people suffering from seasonal affective disorder or SAD, wintertime depression linked to a lack of exposure to sunlight.

Vitamin D deficiency results in progressive hearing loss, thinning of the bones (e.g., osteopenia and osteoporosis), bone deformity (e.g., rickets and osteomalacia), and muscle pain. The body can make its own supply of vitamin D upon exposure to the ultraviolet B rays in sunlight. In fact, an accumulated 45 minutes per week in the midday sunlight (on your face, arms or hands) supplies your body with the "sunshine vitamin" it needs. However, darker skinned people may need more sun exposure than lighter skinned people. If you live in northern latitudes, you'll need to take vitamin D supplements during the months when sunlight is scarce. As you age, your ability to make vitamin D will decline, so check with your doctor for his or her recommendation for additional nutritional supplements—especially if you don't get vitamin D from fortified foods such as milk. The use of sunscreen is an important strategy for reducing the risk of skin cancer, but sunscreen with an SPF 15 can reduce vitamin D production by up to 95 percent.

The most reliable sources of vitamin D are vitamin D-fortified milk and cereals. Other food sources include liver, egg yolk, and fatty fish (e.g., sardines, mackerel, salmon and herring). There is no DV for vitamin D but adults should consume at least 400 IU daily, and people over age 50 may need up to 800 IU daily. Because this nutrient is fat-soluble, vitamin D supplements should be taken after a high-fat meal.

Vitamin E

Vitamin E is a family of eight fat-soluble compounds: namely alpha-, beta-, gamma-, and delta-tocopherols; and alpha-, beta-, gamma-, and delta-tocotrienols. In the past decade, this vitamin has been both praised and vilified. Some studies show significant disease-modulating benefits of vitamin E supplementation while others implicate it in the development of cancer and heart disease. Proponents of vitamin E supplementation charge that the studies showing that vitamin E is detrimental are poorly designed and may be biased. Let's now look at arguments for vitamin E supplementation.

Vitamin E is a component of the membrane that surrounds every cell in the human body, serving an important function in selectively preventing dangerous chemicals from entering the cells and damaging DNA, enzymes, and other important cell structures. Other major functions of vitamin E are to: serve as antioxidants by intercepting free radicals; prevent oxidation of LDL (or so-called "bad") cholesterol; prevent platelets from sticking together (i.e., reduce the formation of abnormal blood clots); and help regulate the function of vitamin A and other nutrients.

Many cardiologists recommend vitamin E as an adjunctive strategy in fighting coronary artery disease. Not surprising since vitamin E prevents LDL cholesterol from oxidizing and platelets from sticking together to form clots. In its oxidized form, LDL cholesterol can stick to blood vessel walls and contribute to arteriosclerosis, the process of developing plaques that narrows blood vessels, putting a person at risk for heart attack and stroke.

Symptoms of vitamin E deficiency include anemia, poor coordination, muscle weakness, and damage to the retina of the eyes. The main food sources of vitamin E include vegetable oils, avocados, whole grain breads and cereals, nuts, broccoli, spinach, and dried prunes. You should get vitamin E primarily from foods but most people will need to take a daily high-potency vitamin supplement, after a high-fat meal.

The DV for vitamin E is 22 IU for adult men and women, but most experts recommend between 200 IU and 400 IU to improve overall health and wellness. I recommend the d-alpha tocopherol which is more biologically active than the synthetic dl-alpha tocopherol. Unlike other fat-soluble vitamins, vitamin E is relatively non-toxic in large amounts. However, large amounts of vitamin E can interfere with the clotting function of vitamin K.

Vitamin K

This fat-soluble vitamin helps with blood clotting. Surgeons use vitamin K before surgery to minimize postoperative bleeding. Besides promoting clotting in the body, vitamin K helps the body use calcium to build strong bones. Recent studies suggest its role in cancer and heart disease prevention.

Signs of deficiency include easy bruising, nose bleeds, and blood in the urine. However, vitamin K deficiency is rare because the body can manufacture most of what it needs. Indeed, approximately 80 percent of the body's vitamin K needs are met through production by friendly intestinal bacteria. Vitamin K is also found in leafy green vegetables, egg yolk, soybean oil, and liver. The DV for this nutrient is 20 to 60 μg but the optimal dose is around 300 μg daily, taken after meals. High doses can be dangerous if you are taking blood thinners such as Coumadin.

Table 3-1

Recommended and Optimal Dosage of Selected Vitamins

Vitamin	Recommended Daily Value	Optimal Daily Dose
A	2,300 IU (women); 3,000 IU (men)	5,000-10,000 (men and women)
B1 (thiamine)	1.5 mg	50-100 mg
B2 (riboflavin)	15 mg	50 mg
B3 (niacin)	14 mg (women); 15 mg (men)	50 mg (men and women)
B5 (pantothenic acid)	None established	100-500 mg
B6 (pyridoxine)	1.3-1.7 mg	50-100 mg
B12 (cyanoco-balamin)	2.4 µg	400-1000 µg
Biotin	None established	35-60 µg
Folic acid	400-600 µg	400-600 µg
C	75 mg (women); 90 mg (men)	200 mg
D	None established	400-800 IU
E	22 IU	200-400 IU
K	20–60 µg	300 µg

MINERALS FROM A TO Z

Like vitamins, minerals are indispensable to health and life. These nutrients are crucial to the basic functions of every cell in the human body, and are needed to build protein, produce energy, and participate in many functions such as muscle contraction and nerve conduction. Unlike vitamins, however, the amount of minerals needed is comparatively miniscule. Minerals can be divided into two groups: the macrominerals and microminerals. The macrominerals that I'll discuss are calcium, chromium, magnesium, phosphorous, silicon, sodium, and sulfur. The micronutrients that I'll discuss are copper, iodine, iron, manganese, molybdenum, potassium, selenium and zinc.

Calcium

Calcium is a mineral that's needed in abundance from cradle to grave. It helps newborns and infants develop strong bones and it lays the groundwork for the first teeth. Adults need calcium to maintain strong bones, healthy teeth, and myriad physiological functions. A small amount of calcium circulates in the blood to help move nutrients across cell membrane and aid in the production of hormones and enzymes that aid in metabolism and digestion. Calcium is also needed for wound healing, muscle contraction and blood clotting.

Calcium plays an important role in regulating the diameter of blood vessels. Not surprisingly, low intake of this mineral has been implicated in elevated blood pressure. Indeed, researchers at McMaster University in Ontario, Canada have linked low daily intake of calcium to the development of high blood pressure.[9] Low calcium intake is also associated with other medical conditions, such as *osteoporosis*, a condition characterized by the leaching of calcium from the bones that eventually makes them thin. This condition is especially prevalent in postmenopausal women with low levels of estrogen. Osteoporosis places a person at risk for hip and other fractures and the resulting complications.

Symptoms of calcium deficiency include muscle spasm, elevated blood pressure, and accelerated bone loss. Calcium can be found in dairy products and in green leafy vegetables. Men and premenopausal women need 1000 mg each per day; after menopause, women need 1500 mg every day. People with thyroid and kidney diseases should check with their doctor before taking calcium supplements.

Chromium

This very popular mineral has many physiological functions. It helps the body metabolize fats, carbohydrates, and proteins. In recent years, chromium has been recognized as a nutrient to help control blood sugar (by enhancing the effects of insulin), and may help control cholesterol levels.

Chromium deficiency presents with impaired glucose tolerance and elevated cholesterol levels. Natural sources of chromium include green beans, broccoli, whole grain products, brewer's yeast, and processed meats. There is no DV established for this nutrient but prominent clinicians recommend up to 200 μg daily to help manage diabetes, high cholesterol, and other problems. Chromium supplements absorb better in the presence of vitamin C.

Copper

Copper is a common micronutrient found mostly in the brain, heart, liver and kidneys. Its major biochemical roles include connective tissue repair, energy production, and the facilitation of mitochondrial and enzyme function. Copper also helps blood to clot and the skin to produce melanin, which maintains normal pigment of the skin and hair. This mineral has also been credited with preventing high blood pressure, heart disease and some cancers. The use of copper bracelets to manage arthritis has produced mixed results.

Wilson's disease, an inherited condition in which the body is unable to rid itself of excess copper, can result in nerve damage and liver failure. Copper deficiency is rare, but when it does occur, symptoms typically include anemia, loss of pigmentation of the hair and skin, impaired cognitive function, and increased susceptibility to infections. Food sources of copper include crabs, lobsters, oysters, liver, legumes, nuts and seeds. There is no DV for this nutrient but adults should take in 1.5 to 3 mg daily. Supplements should be taken after meals to minimize the potential for stomach irritation.

Iodine

Iodine will go down in history as a public health success story. In the 1920s, the US government mandated its addition to table salt as a way to combat widespread deficiency that manifested as thyroid disease and *cretinism*, a form of mental retardation. This strategy resulted in a dramatic lowering of both thyroid diseases and cretinism. As a component of thyroid hormones, iodine is involved in the regulation of gene expression; the rate of metabolism; growth and development; nerve and muscle function; reproductive function; water and electrolyte regulation; and the use of oxygen by cells.

Iodine deficiency can result in thyroid enlargement known as goiter, and eventually an under production of thyroid hormone (a condition called *hypothyroidism*). Since thyroid hormone influences virtually every cell and organ in the body, hypothyroidism can produce a long list of symptoms such as cognitive dysfunction, fatigue, insomnia, dry skin and even death. Besides table salt (which contains 300 μg of iodine per teaspoon), iodine is found in saltwater shellfish, kelp and other sea vegetables. The DV for this mineral is 150 μg daily, with most people in the US getting more than the DV.

Iron

This mineral is an indispensable part of hemoglobin, the pigment in red blood cells that carry oxygen. Indeed, low iron intake can result in iron-deficiency anemia and the body's reduced capacity to transport oxygen. As you know, oxygen is needed by every cell in the body to produce energy, and one of the first signs of iron deficiency is fatigue. Iron also strengthens the immune system, which helps the body to resist germs.

Besides fatigue, iron deficiency results in a rapid heart rate, palpitation, spoon-shaped nails, sores at the corners of the mouth, a sore tongue, and a reduction in size of the taste buds. Iron deficiency is a common problem among menstruating women (due to monthly blood loss) and pregnant women (due to expanded blood volume).

Iron deficiency among men and postmenopausal women usually indicate a serious medical concern. The DV for iron is as follows: for pregnant women, 27 mg; menstruating women, 18 mg; postmenopausal women, 8 mg; and men, 8 mg. Unless recommended by a healthcare professional, men and postmenopausal women should never take supplemental iron due to the risk of heart disease and colon cancer caused by iron overload.

Magnesium

This essential mineral functions as a co-factor in more than 300 biochemical processes such as muscle contraction, nerve function, the formation of bones, and overall metabolism. Low magnesium levels may lead to constriction of blood vessels, which can drive up blood pressure. In fact, researchers at the Harvard University School of Public Health found a correlation between high blood pressure and a low blood magnesium level.[10] Low magnesium can also lead to irregular heartbeat (cardiac arrhythmia). Magnesium has been credited with improving a long list of medical conditions including premenstrual syndrome, fibromyalgia, asthma, type 2 diabetes, and osteoporosis. Unfortunately, magnesium has also been shown to counteract many of the actions of calcium.

The American Dietetic Association estimates that only 50 percent of Americans get the correct amount of magnesium daily. Magnesium deficiency can produce confusion, convulsions, personality changes, muscle spasm, elevated blood pressure, nausea and vomiting. Food sources of this mineral include nuts, beans, bananas, whole grains, shellfish, milk, and green leafy vegetables. The DV for this eclectic mineral is as follows: for adults age 19 to 30, 400 mg for men and 310 mg for women; for people older than age 31, 420 mg for men and 320 mg for women. Excessive magnesium intake can lead to diarrhea and abdominal pain.

Manganese

The full extent of the role of manganese in the human body is still being defined. We do know that manganese plays an important role in cartilage and bone formation and glucose metabolism. Additionally, it is a constituent of some enzymes and an activator of others involved in the metabolism of carbohydrates, proteins, and fats.

Manganese deficiency can result in generalized weakness, seizures, growth retardation, and impaired fertility. Food sources of manganese include nuts, grains, Brussels sprouts, spinach, kelp, pineapple, blueberries, and raisins. There is no DV established for this nutrient but most experts recommend 5 mg daily to optimize health and wellness. Excessive manganese intake can interfere with iron absorption.

Molybdenum

In the body, molybdenum is found mostly in the liver, kidneys, bone, and skin. This trace mineral serves as a co-enzyme in alcohol detoxification by the liver, the formation of sulfur-containing amino acids, and the formation of uric acid. Molybdenum deficiency is rare, but when it occurs, symptoms include anemia, loss of appetite, and weight loss. Natural sources of this mineral include green leafy vegetables, brown rice, millet and legumes. The DV for this nutrient for adults is 45 μg per day but the optimal dose is 250 μg daily.

Phosphorus

Phosphorous is found in every cell in the body. Its major functions include: teaming up with calcium to build strong bones and healthy teeth; joining with fats to form phospholipids, which line all of our cells; helping to maintain the pH balance of the blood; and serving as a co-factor in converting fats, carbohydrates, and proteins into energy.

Phosphorous deficiency is rare, because it is found in many foods of plant and animal origin. Chronic use of anticonvulsants or aluminum-containing antacids can reduce absorption of phosphorous. Conversely, vitamin D can enhance phosphorous absorption. Sources of phosphorous include protein-rich meats, fish, poultry, eggs, and dairy products. The DV and the optimal dose for this nutrient is 700 mg for men and women. Excessive phosphorous intake can inhibit calcium absorption.

Potassium

Potassium is a vital mineral that is necessary for muscles to contract and nerves to fire. Researchers associated with the Veterans Administration Cooperative Study Group found that individuals, especially African-Americans, whose diets were low in potassium, run the risk of higher blood pressure compared with those who consumed adequate amounts of the mineral.[11] This problem is compounded if the diet is high in salt.

Potassium deficiency produces confusion, fatigue, muscle weakness and cramps, and abnormal heart rhythms. Foods high in potassium include bananas, avocados, oranges, tomatoes, dried prunes, raisins, meats and poultry. Baked potato with the skin, lima beans, acorn squash, and spinach also contain potassium. I'm a bit leery about prescribing potassium supplements because too much potassium can result in irregular heart rhythms, a potentially dangerous condition in even healthy individuals. People who require potassium supplementation should only do so under the supervision of a doctor or other qualified healthcare provider. There is no DV for this mineral but most medical experts recommend a daily intake of at least 2,000 mg to 3,000 mg.

Selenium

Found in every cell in the body, selenium is most prevalent in the testes, kidneys, pancreas, liver and spleen. This trace mineral helps convert thyroid hormone from its inactive form (known as T4) to its active form (known as T3). Selenium supports the function of numerous enzymes involved in muscle metabolism, protein transport, and the regeneration of vitamin C. It also serves as an antioxidant, protecting DNA, enzymes, and cell membrane from damage by free radicals. A Chinese study suggests that low consumption of selenium throughout life is associated with lower cognitive scores on mental aptitude tests, even after age, education, and other factors were considered.[12]

Many experts credit selenium for its protection against cancer, stroke, heart disease and macular degeneration. In a study done in Linxian province, China where selenium-depleted soil has been blamed for a high incidence of colon cancer, selenium supplements resulted in impressive reductions of gastrointestinal cancers, heart disease and stroke.[13] In a well-designed study published in the *Journal of the American Medical Association*, in 1996, skin cancer patients given daily selenium supplements were twice as likely to survive their disease compared with their peers not given selenium.

Deficiency in selenium produces deficiency in the enzymes it supports. Symptoms can include muscle weakness, cardiac insufficiency and joint deformity. Brazil nuts, seafood, poultry, meats, and grains are good food sources of selenium. This trace mineral is only needed in small amounts. Selenium toxicity can cause hair loss, muscle cramps, diarrhea, joint pain, and fatigue.

The DV for this nutrient is 55 μg for men and women but the optimal dose is up to 200 μg daily. Selenium and vitamin E work in concert, so be sure to get at least 400 IU on vitamin E daily to maximize the efficacy of selenium.

Silicon

Silicon gain notoriety as a controversial substance used in breast implants. This is unfortunate because silicone is an important nutrient that helps with bone growth and with the health of skin, hair and nail. It is also an important element in the formation of cartilage and connective tissue. Studies credit this mineral with helping to prevent the development of Alzheimer's disease. Food sources of silicon include nuts, seeds, oats, apples, whole grains, leafy green vegetables, and beets. There is no DV established for this nutrient but the optimal dose is 5-20 mg daily.

Sodium

Sodium is one of the three major electrolytes in the body (along with potassium and chloride). This mineral is vilified for its role in the development of high blood pressure, but it is an indispensable nutrient for health and life. Sodium is the main electrolyte outside of the human cell that helps create an electrical gradient across the membrane of each cell. Sodium helps maintain blood volume and blood pressure, and plays a key role in muscle and nerve function. Generally, excessive sodium levels result in excess fluid retention; low sodium levels result in fluid loss. Besides hypertension and associated cardiovascular diseases, excessive sodium is linked to the development of stomach cancer.

Signs of sodium deficiency (from sodium loss or excessive fluid leading to diluted concentration of sodium) include excessive sweating, nausea, diarrhea, and heat exhaustion. Natural sources of sodium include table salt, sea salt, kelp, beets and celery. Artificial sources of sodium include processed meats (e.g., bacon and sausage), canned soups, soy sauce and bouillon cubes. The DV for this nutrient is 500 mg to 2400 mg daily but experts recommend a maximum intake of 1200 to 1500 mg daily.

Sulfur

Sulfur is a constituent of teeth, bones, hair, and collagen and a cofactor in many enzymatic activities. It is involved with the production of bile acid needed for fat absorption and digestion. Sulfur also helps with the conversion of proteins, carbohydrates, and fats into energy.

Since the typical Western diet is high in protein, sulfur deficiency is virtually uncommon. Main sources of sulfur include protein-rich foods such as meat, poultry, fish, eggs and beans. The mineral can also be found in radish, onions, garlic, and kale. There is no DV established for this nutrient.

Zinc

Zinc is an essential trace mineral, found in virtually every cell in the human body. Its role spans everything from augmenting the five senses to sexual maturation, and everything in between. In recent years, scientists have shown that zinc can shorten the duration of the common cold and canker sores. Zinc's other myriad benefits include prevention of macular degeneration, management of inflammatory bowel disease, reducing tinnitus (ringing in the ears) and healing ulcers. Clinicians use zinc to help manage acne, eczema, and psoriasis. In men, low zinc levels have been linked to benign prostatic hypertrophy, a non-cancerous enlargement of the prostate. Adolescent nutritional dwarfism is linked to zinc deficiency.

Zinc deficiency produces anemia, reduced taste, poor appetite, nerve damage, and poor wound healing. Food sources of zinc include poultry, liver, pork, beef, eggs, fish, and oysters. The DV for this nutrient is 8 mg for women and 11 mg for men but higher dosages are needed for specific conditions such as acne and eczema. Pregnant women should get 12 mg daily and breastfeeding women need 13 mg daily. If you use a zinc supplement, try to take it one hour before or two hours after meals—this enhances its absorption.

Table 3-2
Recommended and Optimal Dosage of Selected Minerals

Mineral	Recommended Daily Value	Optimal Daily Dose
Calcium	1,000 mg (men and premenopausal wom-en); 1500 mg (post-menopausal women)	Same as RDA
Chromium	None established	300 mg
Copper	None established	1.5-3 mg
Iodine	150 µg	Same as RDA
Iron	8 mg (men); 8-27 mg (women)	Same as RDA
Magnesium	320-420 mg	Same as RDA
Manganese	NE	5 mg
Molybdenum	45µg	250 µg
Phosphorus	700 mg	Same as RDA
Potassium	None established	2000-3000 mg
Selenium	55 µg	200 µg
Silicon	None established	5-20 mg
Sodium	500-2400 mg	Same as RDA
Sulfur	None established	None Established
Zinc	8 mg (women); 11 mg (Men)	Same as RDA

ACCESSORY SUPPLEMENTS

The list of accessory supplements is quite extensive and seems to grow each day. As I said earlier in this chapter, the precise roles of these compounds are still being defined. More and more, accessory supplements are being adopted for their clinical roles in preventing and mitigating diseases. For example, garlic's anti-inflammatory and lipid-lowering properties make it the ideal adjunctive agent to help mitigate high cholesterol and heart disease. Omega-3 oils are being used to augment drugs used to treat heart disease, high blood pressure, high cholesterol, and eczema. Let's now take a look at ten of the more popular accessory compounds around today: alpha lipoic acid, the bioflavonoids, carnitine, choline, co-enzyme Q-10, the digestive enzymes, garlic, ginger, the omega-3 fatty acids, and turmeric.

Alpha-Lipoic Acid

A recent addition to the dietary supplement armamentarium, alpha-lipoic acid is a powerful antioxidant that was discovered in the 1950s. The unique properties of this fat-soluble compound help the body to increase blood flow to nerves and to support the conduction of nerve impulses. Alpha-lipoic acid works with vitamin B1, vitamin B2, pantothenic acid and niacin to breakdown carbohydrates, protein, and fats to produce energy.

Research during the 1980s and 1990s showed its benefits in helping to control blood sugar and prevent nerve damage in diabetics. Clinicians currently recommend the nutrient for people with *Metabolic Syndrome*. Additional benefits of alpha-lipoic acid include protecting the liver and brain against damage by free radicals. A recent Australian study hints that, by increasing production of acetylcholine in the brain, alpha lipoic acid may improve brain health in Alzheimer's sufferers.[14] Additional research is needed to confirm this preliminary finding. Dr. Bruce Ames, a senior scientist at the University of California at Berkeley showed that alpha-lipoic acid (along with acetyl-L-carnitine) improved memory and energy levels in rats. Dr. Ames expects to duplicate these results in humans.

Food sources of alpha-lipoic acid include liver, brewer's yeast, tomatoes, peas and Brussels sprouts. The dose ranges from 50 mg to 600 mg per day. Daily intake over 100 mg should be divided into three doses. This supplement should be taken after a high-fat meal to facilitate absorption.

Potential side effects of alpha-lipoic acid include stomach upset, overstimulation, and insomnia. High doses may cause blood sugar levels to drop too low.

Bioflavonoids

The bioflavonoids (also referred to as flavonoids) are a large family of over 5,000 phytochemicals (plant derivatives) found in the pigment of fruits and vegetables. These naturally occurring, water-soluble nutrients can be categorized as isoflavons (e.g., genistein in soybeans); anthocyanidins (e.g., cyaniding in blueberries); flavanols (e.g., catechin in green tea); flavonols (e.g., quercetin in grapes and garlic); flavones (e.g., apigenin in parsley); and flavanones (e.g., hesperitin in oranges and grapefruits). Because the body cannot produce bioflavonoids, they must be obtained from either foods or supplements.

These compounds are felt to possess antiviral, antihistamine, anticancer, anti-inflammatory, and antioxidant properties. Bioflavonoids have been credited with promoting good health and helping to attenuate and manage a long list of conditions, such as: modulation of estrogen fluctuations; reduction of menopausal symptoms (e.g., anxiety, mood swings, and hot flashes); keeping the skin healthy; and reducing the symptoms of hay fever. In addition, these compounds are felt to strengthen capillaries (small blood vessels), reduce inflammation and lower high cholesterol and high blood pressure. In the body, bioflavonoids help prevent the destruction of vitamin C by oxidation.

Sources of bioflavonoids include blackberries, cherries, grapes, lemons, oranges, and plums. Soy products and green tea are also good sources of flavonoids. There are no side effects of bioflavonoids except reported cases of low-grade fever and hives with catechin. Excessively high doses may cause diarrhea. For best results, bioflavonoids should be combined with vitamin C. There is no DV for bioflavonoids but most natural medicine authorities recommend between 50 mg and 500 mg of mixed bioflavonoids, daily.

Carnitine

Carnitine is derived from the amino acid lysine. Available as D-carnitine, L-carnitine, and DL-carnitine, this nutrient is involved in carbohydrates and protein metabolism. It also helps transport free fatty acids through mitochondrial inner-membranes to facilitate the synthesis of adenosine triphosphate or ATP, the energy package that gives us the strength to perform every living function from breathing to running.

Through its action in facilitating fat burning for energy, carnitine helps lower cholesterol and triglycerides levels, thus preventing heart disease and stroke. Some medical practitioners use this nutrient to help restore energy in people suffering from chronic fatigue syndrome and fibromyalgia, conditions characterized by profound, unremitting fatigue. Other health-promoting and disease-preventing roles of carnitine include slowing of the aging process, improving muscle strength in people with such conditions as muscular dystrophy, and improving the motility of sperm. As I discussed earlier under "Alpha Lipoic Acid," Dr. Bruce Ames, a senior scientist at Children's Hospital Oakland Research Institute in California showed that a combination of acetyl-L-carnitine and alpha lipoic acid improved memory and energy levels in rats—findings he expects to duplicate in humans.

Food sources of carnitine include meats, poultry, fish and dairy products. There are no reported toxic side effects of this nutrient but excess quantities may cause nausea, abdominal cramps, restlessness and insomnia. There is no established DV for carnitine but most experts recommend between 500 mg and 2000 mg/day of the L-carnitine form of the nutrient.

Choline

Classified as a natural food component, choline is an essential nutrient needed to make healthy cell membrane and to support brain development and liver function. Choline transports fats away from the liver preventing the development of a fatty liver. Additionally, it is a precursor to acetylcholine, an important brain chemical involved in preserving memory. Scientific evidence credits choline with lowering blood levels of homocysteine, an amino acid linked to inflammation, heart disease and stroke.

Food sources of choline include egg yolks, legumes, soybeans, milk, meats, peanuts, and green peas. Choline supplements come is a number of different forms such as choline bitartrate, choline chloride, and choline citrate. Side effects of choline supplements include nausea, increased body temperature and excessive sweating. There is no DV for this nutrient but the Linus Pauling Institute recommends a daily intake of 550 mg of choline bitartrate or choline chloride for men and 425 mg for women, after meals.

Co-enzyme Q-10

Produced in the mitochondria of every one of the 100 trillion cells in the body, co-enzyme Q-10 (CoQ10) is indispensable for health and life. Also referred to as ubiquinone to emphasize its widespread distribution in the body, it is not considered a vitamin because the body is able to make it from food. CoQ10 is a fat-soluble nutrient that helps the mitochondria burn carbohydrates and fat to make adenosine triphosphate or ATP, the energy package that gives us the strength to perform every living function from breathing to running.

This world-renowned nutrient is a powerful antioxidant that has been shown to enhance immune function. CoQ10 is credited with an impressive list of health benefits, including: improvement in asthma and hay fever; reduction of migraines; improvement in heart failure; protection of the heart from the damaging effects of blood pressure-lowering, anti-cancer and anti-cholesterol drugs; reduction of blood pressure; and treatment of periodontal disease. Other health conditions for which CoQ10 might help manage include diabetes, muscle wasting disease, immune dysfunction, and cancer. Dr. David Perlmutter, a well-respected neurologist and director of the Perlmutter Health Center in Naples, Florida, believes that CoQ10 deficiency is a major cause of decline in mental function in midlife and degenerative brain diseases, such as Alzheimer's disease, later in life.

As we age, our production of CoQ10 wanes, making supplementation with this nutrient a wise healthy-aging strategy. The statin drugs (such as atorvastatin, lovastatin, simvastatin and rosuvastatin), used to treat high cholesterol, can impair the body's ability to produce adequate amounts of CoQ10. In fact, severe side effects from the statin drugs, such as rhabdomyolysis and heart muscle weakness, are believed to be linked to a drastic drop in CoQ10 levels. Therefore, statin users should supplement with 100 to 200 mg of CoQ10, after meals, daily. The usual daily dose is 30 mg to 60 mg. Food sources of this nutrient include peanuts, spinach, sardines, and liver. If you chose to take a CoQ10 supplement, take it after meals for better absorption.

Digestive Enzymes

Enzymes serve as catalysts to help drive the thousands of biochemical events that take place in the body. Digestive enzymes are produced in the salivary glands and the pancreas to help digest and absorb carbohydrates, protein, and fats. Digestive enzymes supplements are used by individuals with digestive enzyme deficiency to help digest foods and adsorb nutrients from the gastrointestinal tract.

The best known digestive enzyme deficiency is lactase, most common among people of Mediterranean and African descents. Indeed, 80 percent of African Americans and 53 percent of Mexican Americans are lactase deficient. In recent years, some experts suggest that people might have other unrecognized digestive enzyme deficiencies. It stands to reason that the body is unlikely to experience only lactase deficiency and that other deficiencies likely exist. For instance, *leaky gut syndrome* is a condition in which undigested protein seeps through the intestinal wall into the blood stream, creating an allergic reaction. This condition and others should be diagnosed by qualified healthcare professionals.

Other digestive enzymes and their digestive functions include: amylase (complex carbohydrates); bromelain (protein); cellulase (fiber); lipase (fats); maltase (disaccharide); papain (protein); and sucrase (starches). Most digestive enzyme supplements contain the full complements of these catalysts. There are no reported side effects of these products. For best results, take one supplement tablet at the start of each meal.

Garlic

This herb, a member of the family of allium vegetables, has gained culinary and medicinal prominence in multiple cultures over many centuries. Hippocrates, the father of medicine, prescribed garlic for numerous conditions including toothache and leprosy. Today, it is regarded by many conventional and alternative medicine clinicians, medical researchers, and herbalists as a super herb for its litany of health benefits. Garlic's benefits are derived from its many *organosulfur compounds*, which have been shown to: lower cholesterol and triglycerides; reduce the clumping of platelets (which reduces blood clots); reduce inflammation; serve as antioxidants; and inhibit the development of cancer.

According to a 7-year study done at the University of California at Los Angeles, aged garlic extract can benefit people at risk for heart disease.[15] In the study of 3000 individuals, garlic inhibited calcified plaque formation, lowered LDL cholesterol and increased HDL cholesterol. In a randomized, double-blind study of healthy men and women done at East Carolina University School of Medicine in Greenville, North Carolina, garlic extract was shown to inhibit to clumping of platelets, which reduces the risk of blood clots—a major event during a heart attack or stroke.[16]

In another study done in Nittendorf, Germany, garlic was found to significantly lower mild elevations in blood pressure, probably through one of its components methyl allyl trisulfide, which dilates blood vessels. Garlic also contains methylsulfonylmethane, or MSM, an organic sulfur compound that has been shown to reduce inflammation in people with arthritis. MSM also nourishes the skin, hair and nails. Finally, garlic contains antiviral, antifungal, and antibacterial properties, which can be used to help manage the common cold, athlete's foot, and skin infections.

This herb is available as fresh bulbs, oil-based extracts, dried powder, steam-distilled extracts and pills. Adverse effects of garlic include a pungent breath and body odor (due to its sulfur-containing compounds), heartburn, nausea, gas, and diarrhea. Most commercially sold garlic pills are odorless. You can minimize garlic's pungent breath odor by chewing sprigs of parsley or mint. Pregnant women should exercise caution when taking high doses of garlic as it has been shown to stimulate uterine contractions in animal studies. Garlic may impair thyroid function in people with reduced thyroid function. The recommended dose of garlic is 600 to 900 mg daily.

Ginger

This herb has been an ancient favorite in Southeast Asia for thousands of years for its flavoring and medicinal properties. In recent years, healthy aging enthusiasts and natural health practitioners in the West have embraced ginger (Zingiber officinale) as a superstar nutrient. The rhizome (root) of the plant contains a long list of phytochemicals and vitamins that provide numerous health benefits, such as fighting nausea associated with morning-sickness, motion sickness, and chemotherapy, combating inflammatory, and helping to heal sores. Ginger is also used for indigestion and to prevent intestinal gas.

Ginger comes in many forms including dried root, fresh root, tablets, capsules, liquid extract, tincture and tea. This herb is very safe with the most common side effect being stomach upset, which can be minimized by taking ginger tablets instead of powder. Contraindications to using ginger include pregnancy, diabetes, gallstones, heart disease, bleeding disorder, and concurrent use of blood thinners. Most herbalists and other natural health experts recommend between 1000 mg to 4000 mg of ginger daily.

Omega-3 fatty acids

To begin with, omega-3 fatty acids are classified as *essential*, which means that our bodies cannot synthesize them, so we must get them from foods or supplements. These fats—eicosapentaenoic acid (EPA), docosahexaenoic acid (DHA) and alpha-linolenic acid (ALA)—are classified as polyunsaturated and regarded as "healthy fats." They form the basis of cell membranes—including the cells in the brain—and thus are instrumental in selectively admitting nutrients into and out of cells. Much has been written about the wide range of health benefits of the omega-3 fats in helping to mitigate and manage a long list of disorders such as inflammation, blood coagulation, central nervous system (brain) disorders, diabetes, and heart disease.

A large body of scientific evidence shows that omega-3 fatty acids improve the inner structure and function of blood vessels and increase the production of nitric acid, which keeps blood vessels dilated and pliable. These actions are important to lowering blood pressure. Indeed, the omega-3 fatty acids are excellent adjuncts in the management of high blood pressure. These healthy fats also reduce a person's risk for heart disease by increasing HDL (so-called, "good") cholesterol and decreasing LDL (so-called, "bad") cholesterol and triglycerides levels. Additionally, the omega-3 fatty acids help prevent irregular heart beats by supporting the function of the heart's electrical circuitry.

The omega-3 fats also lower levels of arachidonic acid, a major player in the development of inflammation and pain. In fact, many clinicians prescribe omega-3 fatty acids to help manage arthritis and other inflammatory conditions. A number of studies suggest that these fats can attenuate symptoms of depression (including post-partum depression in women); suicide; attention deficit hyperactivity disorder (ADHD); and migraine headaches. Other suggested benefits include reducing the risk for prostate and breast cancers; improving lung function in asthma; and reducing the symptoms of painful menstruation.

There is also some conflicting evidence (I believe, due to poor study design) that these fats don't deliver the benefits uncovered by many studies. At any rate, the Food and Drug Administration allows food manufacturers to make the following claim about the omega-3 fatty acids: "Supportive but not conclusive research shows that consumption of EPA and DHA omega-3 fatty acids may reduce the risk of coronary heart disease." The American Heart Association recommends the use of omega-3 fats to help prevent heart disease. I believe that most adults and children should supplement their diet with an omega-3 supplement every day.

Although food should be the primary source of nutrients, some authorities, such as esteemed integrative medicine physician, Dr. Andrew Wei, believe that fish oil supplements might be superior to dietary sources of omega-3 fats. Some food sources of these fats, such as salmon and tuna, contain toxic levels of mercury, dioxin and PCBs (polychlorinated biphenyls). Fish oil supplements from reputable sources are purified and free of toxic elements. Another reason to take fish oil supplements is that other sources of omega-3 fats, such as walnuts, flaxseed, canola oil and soybeans, don't contain EPA and DHA but rather a precursor element that the body has to convert to EPA and DHA. The conversion process is variable between persons and can be inhibited by factors such as trans-fats found in fast foods.

The recommended daily intake of omega-3 fats is between 1000 mg and 2000 mg for health maintenance. People with diabetes, heart disease, migraine headaches, ADHD, and other conditions may need 3000 mg per day. Doses higher than 3000 mg per day should be taken only under medical supervision due to the risk of excessive thinning of the blood. Because EPA and DHA are fat-soluble, you should take them after a meal containing some fat to optimize absorption.

Turmeric

Turmeric (*curcuma longa*), an ancient plant native to India that dates back 4000 years, has become a perennial favorite of people interested in the natural approach to healthcare. Curcumin, the phytochemical substance that gives turmeric its yellow color, has been credited with numerous health benefits, such as ameliorating the symptoms of arthritis, strengthening heart function, and helping to beat back cancer. This powerful antioxidant also has antiviral, antibacterial, and antiparasitic properties. In India and China, turmeric is used topically in creams and ointments to treat eczema and ringworm.

Turmeric is very safe with no reported side effects with recommended doses. Contraindications to using turmeric include pregnancy and a history of gallstones. People taking anticoagulants (blood thinners) should avoid turmeric as it might add to the blood thinning effects of anticoagulants. Most herbalists and other natural health experts recommend between 250 mg and 500 mg of turmeric three times daily.

WHICH SUPPLEMENTS ARE RIGHT FOR YOU?

So many supplements, so little time! There's so much evidence for and so much evidence against the routine use of dietary supplements. How's the average person supposed to decide? In my wellness practice, I almost always recommend supplements for my patients based on their individual need. I recommend a multivitamin/multimineral supplement for basic health and wellness maintenance for people without health problems. For my patients with health problems, I recommend a combination of various vitamins, minerals, and accessory nutrients.

My recommendations are based on my piecing together recommendations by various experts in health promotion and disease prevention. Doses vary from person-to-person and for different diseases. Drug-supplement interaction is becoming a major problem for people concurrently taking drugs and supplements, so before combining drugs and supplements check with your healthcare provider. Let's now examine my recommendations for health maintenance supplements and disease-fighting supplements (also delineated in Table 3-3).

Table 3-3

Supplements for Health Maintenance and Disease Fighting

Supplements for Health Maintenance

- Pharmaceutical-grade multivitamin/mineral supplement
- An antioxidant (Vitamins C and E, co-enzyme Q-10, and selenium)
- Digestive enzymes (amylase, bromelain, cellulase lipase, maltase, papain, and sucrase)

Supplements that Fight Disease

- Alpha lipoic acid and chromium
- Folate
- Omega-3 fatty acids
- Co-enzyme Q-10
- Bioflavonoid with vitamin C.
- Miscellaneous supplements (garlic, ginger, turmeric, and L-carnitine)

Supplements for Health Maintenance

To protect against chronic disease, fill nutritional gaps, and to manage the aging process, I believe that most people should take a pharmaceutical-grade multivitamin/multimineral supplement after a high-fat meal, everyday. This is especially true as you get older and your cells and organs become less efficient at carrying out the thousands of biochemical processes needed for life and optimal health.

The Antioxidants. A lion share of the literature on dietary supplements in the past decade has been about the antioxidant supplements. These represent a group of nutrients—e.g., Vitamins C and E, co-enzyme Q-10, and selenium—that guard against *free radicals*, which are toxic by-products produced in the body as a results of normal metabolism. Free radicals are toxic to the body because, unlike normal molecules, they exist as unpaired (and unstable) electrons that steal electrons from other sources to create even pairs. Antioxidants donate electrons to free radicals to even them up and to render them stable.

Left unchecked, free radicals steal electrons from cell membranes, DNA, and enzymes, damaging these vital structures and starting disease processes. Indeed, these pesky elements are felt to be the basis for most chronic diseases (e.g., heart disease, diabetes, and cancer) as well as the process of accelerated aging. Fortunately, the body produces its own antioxidants—two enzymes called superoxide dismutase and catalase.

Despite the fact that the body produces its own antioxidants and my belief that the best sources of exogenous antioxidants are fresh fruits and vegetables, I recommend that most of my patients take a daily antioxidant supplement. Why? First, most people don't consume the recommended 5 to 10 servings of fruits and vegetables everyday. Secondly, excessive emotional stress, environmental pollutants, unhealthy foods, and other factors expose the average person to excessive amounts of free radicals that can overwhelm the body's antioxidant system. Lastly, as we age, we become less efficient at absorbing nutrients (including vitamins) from foods. As we age, also, our superoxide dismutase production wanes, leaving us vulnerable to the ravages of free radicals.

It is important to consume both fat-soluble and water-soluble antioxidants. The fat-soluble agents, like vitamin E, can penetrate the cell and neutralize free radicals that are produced within the cell. On the other hand, the water-soluble vitamins, such as vitamin C, can't penetrate the cell but can work on free radicals outside the cell.

Digestive Enzymes. I recommend the routine use of digestive enzymes, under doctors' supervision, for people with known digestive enzyme deficiency and for those with chronic gastrointestinal conditions. Persons with lactase deficiency (the largest group being African Americans) probably have other digestive enzyme deficiency and should take a multi-enzyme dietary supplement that contains amylase, bromelain, cellulase lipase, maltase, papain, and sucrase. You should also take a multi-enzyme supplement if you've had other gastrointestinal problems such as irritable bowel syndrome, Crohn's disease, ulcerative colitis and gastroesophageal reflux disease. People who have undergone gastric by-pass surgery and those with malabsorption problems should also take a multi-enzyme supplement.

Supplements that Fight Disease

As I mentioned earlier, the role of nutritional supplements in ameliorating and managing disease is rapidly coming into sharp focus. That folic acid significantly lowers a woman's risk of giving birth to a child with neural tube defect is only the tip of the iceberg in terms of adopting dietary supplements to help fight disease. More evidence of the disease-fighting benefits of nutritional supplements is bound to emerge in the coming years.

Alpha Lipoic Acid & Chromium. These two agents are a must-have for the millions of Americans with diagnosed and undiagnosed metabolic syndrome and diabetes. Again, they combine to help fight insulin resistance and normalize blood sugar levels. Chromium also has an important role in helping to convert the inactive form of thyroid hormone to its active form. Therefore, if you suffer from hypothyroidism (an under-active thyroid gland), you should ask your doctor about supplementing your regular treatment with daily chromium.

Folate/Folic Acid. Women of childbearing age who wish to conceive, should take folate, daily—starting months before they become pregnant. As discussed earlier, this member of the B-vitamin family is credited with a dramatic fall in incidence of birth defect of the brain and spinal cord among newborns. Folic acid also lowers the blood levels of homocysteine, an amino acid linked to the development of heart disease. I predict that lowering homocysteine levels in the blood will become a routine strategy for preventing heart disease, similar to our approach to lowering cholesterol.

The Omega-3 Fatty Acids. As I discussed earlier under "Accessory Supplements," emerging evidence is beginning to credit these essential fats with mitigating a long list of diseases. Based on current evidence, I believe that people with any brain condition such as ADD/ADHD, migraine headache, Parkinson's disease, Alzheimer's disease, and depression should consume between 2000 mg and 3000 mg of omega-3 fatty acids, daily. This also goes for individuals with heart disease and inflammatory conditions such as gouty arthritis, osteoarthritis and rheumatoid arthritis.

Co-enzyme Q-10. After age 40 or so, the body produces less and less co-enzyme Q-10. Therefore, most people older than 40 years-old should also take coenzyme Q-10 after a high-fat meal, daily. This is absolutely necessary if you are taking one of the cholesterol lowering drugs such as atorvastatin, lovastatin, simvastatin and rosuvastatin, which have been shown to deplete the body's co-enzyme Q-10 levels. Other conditions that this superstar nutrient might help treat include high blood pressure, heart failure, migraine headache, chronic fatigue syndrome, fibromyalgia, and arthritis. Doses vary, so check with a qualified healthcare professional for the dose that's right for you.

Bioflavonoids. As discussed above, these plant-based nutrients offer a wide array of health benefits and more benefits are being discovered. People with hay fever and asthma might do well with a bioflavonoid supplement that includes quercetin combined with vitamin C.

Miscellaneous Supplements. Other supplements to consider include garlic, ginger, turmeric, and L-carnitine. These compounds provide an eclectic range of health benefits, the extent of which is predicted to expand precipitously as scientific research illuminates their disease-fighting and health-promoting properties.

Which Forms of Supplements are Best?

As I mentioned earlier, supplements come in pills, capsules, liquids, and powder forms. Some people do better with capsules, others prefer liquids. Considerations include: the ability to swallow certain forms of a product; whether or not the product leaves an after taste; and whether or not the product upsets your stomach.

I recommend that you select the form that is easiest for you to take. If you develop nausea or abdominal pain after taking your supplements, I'd recommend you discontinue all your supplements for a few days. Then restart your supplements one at a time, with two or three days between reintroduction of each supplement. Stop the supplement that causes abdominal distress. Some people are able to tolerate a different form of the same supplement. For example, if the capsule form of a given supplement induces nausea, the pill form of the same supplement might be completely tolerable.

HOW TO FIND HIGH-QUALITY DIETARY SUPPLEMENTS

The nutritional supplement industry is predicted to be a $35B a year business by 2010, with thousands of small and large manufacturers competing for these dollars. These products are sold in supermarkets, pharmacies, health food stores, doctor's offices, and via network marketing. One of the most common questions I get in my wellness practice is: How and where do I find high-quality dietary supplements?

There is no question: the manufacture and distribution of dietary supplements remain an enigma to the most sophisticated consumer. Criticisms leveled at the nutrition supplements industry include a lack of regulation by the Food and Drug Administration (FDA). Indeed, the Dietary Supplement Health and Education Act passed by Congress in 1994 places the burden of proof of product potency on the FDA, not the manufacturer. As you can imagine, some unscrupulous companies have exploited this loophole in the law and are producing sub-par products. Unfortunately, this has given a bad name to the entire industry, and has provided ammunition to critics bent on vilifying the routine use of these health-promoting, disease-preventing products.

A high-quality product meets the following standards: it is potent, bioavailable, and meets good manufacturing practice (GMP) as delineated by the FDA. What does all this mean? Potency means a supplement contains the product and the amount it advertises. Bioavailability has to do with the product's ability to absorb via the gastrointestinal tract into the bloodstream and into the cells. GMP requires that the supplement maker adheres to quality systems and procedures of designing, manufacturing, packaging, labeling and storing the product.

In-house quality control practices are good, but independent quality control testing is the gold standard. Nutritional supplements that bear the GMP seal of the Natural Products Association meet the industry benchmark for potency, bioavailability, and GMP. NPA's contact information is listed in Appendix I.

IN SUMMARY

- Vitamins, minerals and other micronutrients are indispensable to each and every biochemical function of the body. These nutrients also protect the body from free radicals and other dangerous elements. Emerging scientific evidence show that micronutrients also fight diseases such as cancer, high blood pressure, and hay fever.
- Fruits and vegetables should be the primary source of micronutrients. However, less than 30 percent of Americans get these essential nutrients from their diet, making dietary supplements a necessary alternative for most people. Other factors that make dietary supplementation a necessary health and wellness strategy are: our nutrient-depleted foods, toxic environments, and the biologic inefficiency of the aging body.
- To enhance adsorption of the fat-soluble nutrients, take your supplements after meals.
- Look for products that are potent and bioavailable, and meet good manufacturing practices.

Chapter 4

Engage in Daily Physical Activity

"All parts of the body which have a function, if used in moderation and exercised in labors to which each is accustomed, become healthy and well developed and age slowly. But if used and left idle, they become liable to disease, defective in growth and age quickly."
—Hippocrates, 370 B.C.

Plain and simple: The human body was meant to be moved! When it comes to our various organ systems, the old adage "use it or lose it" aptly applies. It's quite fascinating to know that this is very old knowledge, recognized as far back as the 3rd millennia. All of our organs, including muscles, the brain, the heart, the kidneys, and the liver need to be in a state of dynamic flux, which is largely facilitated by regular physical activity.

Sadly, 60 percent of Americans don't get the recommended daily amount of exercise, and 25 percent are not active at all. How did we become such a sedentary society? Did anyone see this coming? What do we do now?

The flip side of the impressive technological advances of the last millennium (e.g., improvements in workplace efficiency and nifty household amenities such as the TV remote control) is that we've developed perfect strategies for pursuing *physical inactivity*. Indeed, our technological successes have spawned a *sedentary mindset* and a litany of sedentary-induced lifestyle diseases. Experts declare that most chronic diseases that plague Americans today are directly or indirectly attributable to physical inactivity. We are currently at the crossroads of our impressive advancements: we are now paying dearly for self-induced physical inertia and we are beginning to examine the paradox of modern living.

THE HIGH PRICE OF PHYSICAL INACTIVITY

You can't achieve wellness while pursuing a sedentary lifestyle! Physical inactivity leads to a long list of health conditions: depression, anxiety and excessive stress; impaired cognitive function; overweight and obesity; cardiovascular disease; diabetes; osteoporosis; and some types of cancer. In fact, the Centers for Disease Control and Prevention (CDC) estimates that physical inactivity along with poor nutrition is responsible for 300,000 *preventable* deaths among Americans each year!

Let's now examine each sedentary-induced health condition and how they occur and, in the next section, we'll discuss ways to prevent and fix each problem.

Depression and Anxiety

People who lead sedentary lives are more prone to psychological diseases compared to their physically active peers. A study published in 2008 in the journal *General Hospital Psychiatry*, researchers linked physical inactivity to depression, anxiety and obesity.[1]

Impaired Cognitive Function

Physical activity enhances cognitive abilities, especially as you get older. On the other hand, physical inertia negatively impacts the functional integrity of the brain (planning, organizing and working memory). When the body is sedentary there is reduced blood flow to the brain. Less blood means less oxygen, an indispensible catalyst for virtually all brain function. A 10-year study of men from Finland, Italy, and the Netherlands showed that the cognitive decline among participants who reduced their daily physical activity by an hour or more was 2.6 times greater that their peers who maintained the same level of physical activity.

Overweight and Obesity

A sedentary lifestyle is a major risk factor for overweight and obesity. Physical inactivity doubles ones risk of developing overweight and obesity. Health experts declare that physical inertia is one of the major reasons why 65 percent of Americans today exceed their ideal body weight.

Cardiovascular Disease

A lack of exercise is a significant risk factor for cardiovascular disease—i.e., stroke, heart disease and high blood pressure. The American Heart Association estimates that sedentary individuals are twice as likely to develop cerebral and coronary artery diseases, which can lead to stroke and heart attack.[2] Additionally, a sedentary lifestyle imposes a 30 to 50 percent risk of developing high blood pressure. Indeed, the majority of hypertensive individuals report physical inactivity as one of the risk factors for developing this condition.

Diabetes

Physical inactivity has spawned an epidemic of type 2 diabetes among Americans—both adults and children. Type 2 diabetes, traditionally regarded as adult-onset diabetes, now affects a record-number of children and adolescents. The incidence of this disease among adults has also skyrocketed. Type 2 diabetes is predicted to impose a spectacular disease burden on our society in the coming years.

Osteoporosis

Osteoporosis, the thinning of bones that predisposes a person to fractures, is a common and expensive disease. The National Osteoporosis Foundation estimates that 10 million Americans suffer from this condition and 34 million more are at risk for developing it.[3] Osteoporosis and its complications cost our society $19B to treat annually.

Epidemiological studies link a sedentary lifestyle as a primary driver of this disease. It seems that weight-bearing physical activity is more important than calcium, magnesium and vitamin D in building bone density. In fact, osteoporosis is most prevalent in countries with the highest calcium consumption. Astronauts in weightless flight develop osteoporosis very quickly.

Cancer

Although genetic endowment is responsible for some cases of cancer, the American Cancer Society estimates that the vast majority of cancer cases each year are attributed to modifiable behaviors such as unhealthy eating and physical inactivity.[4] Scientists have linked physical inactivity and a sedentary lifestyle to the development of cancers of the colon, breasts, and prostate.

Premature Death

Solid scientific evidence shows that physical inactivity increases the risk of premature death (i.e., dying earlier than the average age of death for a given population). Sedentary individuals generally have higher rates of heart disease, stroke, cancer, diabetes, osteoporosis, arthritis, depression, anxiety, and mental decline compared with their physically active peers. Physical inactivity is such a high predictor of mortality that it trumps any protection ethnicity, gender or genetic endowment might bestow.

THE BENEFITS OF PHYSICAL ACTIVITY

Physical activity can influence the way we age. The American College of Sports Medicine, the American Heart Association, and other health and fitness advocates recognize physical activity as an integral part of health, wellness and healthy aging. Dr. Ronald Klatz of the

National Academy of Sports Medicine says that "exercise is strong medicine." In fact, it has been shown that aerobic exercise (e.g., walking, jogging, swimming, dancing, gardening, and hiking) can be as effective as drugs in lowering mild high blood pressure, high cholesterol and triglycerides, and high blood sugar! Needless to say, exercise is cheaper than drugs and doesn't incur the risk of side effects caused by many medications.

People who exercise on a regular basis report better physical, emotional, social and spiritual health than their sedentary peers. Indeed, the CDC reports that regular physical activity produces a wide range of health benefits, including the prevention and mitigation of the most common chronic diseases that affect Americans today. Moreover, active individuals are less likely to die prematurely when compared to their inactive peers. Let's now examine how exercise can keep you healthy and well:

Mental and Emotional Health

Physically active people are less prone to psychological diseases compared to their physically inactive peers. In a 1999 study published in the *Archives of Internal Medicine*, modest physical activity effectively lowered the incidence of depression, anxiety and excessive stress among men and women. Physical exertion burns up negative hormones and neurotransmitters like adrenaline and cortisol and enhances the production of beneficial molecules such as dopamine, serotonin, and endorphins.

Cognitive Function

Physical activity increases blood flow and oxygen to the brain, facilitating the mobilization and activity of the brain's neurotransmitters, the substances the brain uses to relay information between brain cells. Neurobiologists have demonstrated that the production and actions of dopamine, serotonin and other neurotransmitters correlate with cognitive function.

Body Weight

If you exceed your ideal weight, regular physical activity can help you achieve a healthy weight. Medical scientists at the University of Maryland, School of Medicine discovered that exercise can modify the so-called "obesity gene" or FTO thereby preventing weight gain in carriers of this gene.

Cardiovascular Health

Dr. Dean Ornish and others have demonstrated in impressive research that regular physical activity can help reverse cardiovascular disease. Aerobic exercise raises blood HDL cholesterol (i.e., the so-called good cholesterol), and lowers the so-called bad or LDL cholesterol, and triglycerides.

Regular aerobic exercise also strengthens your cardiovascular (heart and blood vessel) system and contributes to overall well-being. A stronger heart leads to improved cardiac output, which means the heart pumps more blood and performs more efficiently with each beat. In other words, physical exertion makes your heart a stronger muscle, forces you to breathe deeply, and provides more oxygen to the lungs, heart muscle, brain, and the rest of the body.

Physical activity has been shown to effectively reduce the risk of developing high blood pressure and to manage high blood pressure if you already are hypertensive. The American College of Sports Medicine recently evaluated 40 scientific studies and found that aerobic exercise done 20 minutes or more three to five days a week can reduce both systolic and diastolic blood pressures by an average of 10 mm Hg.[5] This can help you avoid a dangerous disease and the burden of taking expensive drugs (and their side effects) every day for the rest of your life.

Building Strong Bones

A most important strategy for preventing and treating osteoporosis is weight-bearing physical activities (e.g., walking, jogging and dancing) and non-weight-bearing exercise (e.g., weight lifting, using exercise elastic bands and lifting your own weight). The National Osteoporosis Foundation recommends that all adults engage in 30 minutes of weight bearing exercise most days of the week and resistance/strengthening exercise two to three days per week. For resistance exercise, work most major muscles (upper, middle and lower back; shoulder and upper arms; chest; abdominals; thighs; and calves). Do one or two sets of 8 to 10 repetitions of each exercise.

Cancer Prevention

Physical activity is one of your best defenses against cancer—a disease predicted to affect 50 percent of Americans. In a scientific study published in the highly-regarded *British Medical Journal*, breast cancer patients who exercised regularly at moderate levels had better quality of life indices (i.e., functional and psychological capacity) than their sedentary counterparts.[6]

The American Cancer Society recommends that all adults engage in at least 30 minutes of moderate to vigorous physical activity—above usual activities—on five or more days per week.[4] These activities can include walking, jogging, dancing, and swimming.

Healthy Aging and Longevity

The health research literature is clear: physically active people live healthier and longer lives than their sedentary peers. Physically active individuals generally have lower rates of heart disease, stroke, cancer, diabetes, osteoporosis, arthritis, depression, anxiety, and mental decline compared with their sedentary peers. Physical activity—even low-level activity—imparts a huge measure of protection that trumps any disease- and mortality-enhancing challenges imposed by ethnicity, gender or genetic endowment.

Other Health Benefits of Physical Activity

Regular physical activity provides other important health benefits. Compared to their sedentary peers, persons who engage in regular exercise report enhanced self-confidence, opportunity for socializing, better muscle tone and strength, increased lean body mass, improved digestion, improved sleep quality, and overall good health and well-being.

Emerging evidence points to better hormonal balance among women who engage in regular physical activity. Finally, exercise helps prevent falls among the elderly by mitigating age-related decline in muscle strength, joint function, core strength, inner ear function, and brain function.

BARRIERS TO PHYSICAL ACTIVITY

There are very few *legitimate* barriers to physical activity but many *perceived* barriers. Real barriers include physical disability, severe cardiovascular disease, and environmental constraints such as crime and lack of facilities. Clearly, people with disabling arthritis, those with uncontrolled angina, and individuals rendered home-bound due to crime have valid challenges when it comes to pursuing an exercise program. These people should work with their healthcare provider to achieve optimal management of their disease and to discuss at-home options.

Well-Worn Excuses

Perhaps the most common reason people fail to exercise is the list of excuses they develop for not exercising. Some of the more common excuses for not exercising include:

- "I'm too busy."
- "It's dark during the time I can exercise."
- "It's raining."
- "My feet hurt."
- "I'm in poor physical shape."
- "I'm too old."
- "I can't afford to."

In my clinical experience, people will always find the time to do the things they *perceive* as important. Therefore, the above list of excuses is formulated via a mindset that doesn't place physical activity high on a priority list. Considering that a good exercise program takes only about 150 minutes each week, everyone's schedule can accommodate a few 30-minute exercise sessions per week. Whether it's less time watching TV or talking on the telephone, *everyone* can find time to exercise.

Walking at lunchtime is one way to get around the excuse of "not enough daylight time." You should have an indoor exercise program—such as a stationary bike—for days when inclement weather precludes outside activity or when short winter days preclude outdoor exercises during evening hours.

For the most part, poor physical shape is not a valid excuse. With proper screening by your doctor and a clear exercise prescription, even individuals in poor physical health can engage in a graduated exercise program. However, you have to stop making excuses and take the first step—today!

As we age, our level of physical activity drops off. However, aging and most physical impairments are not barriers to exercising. New research indicates that healthy people in their 70s and 80s can safely undertake physically appropriate exercises on a regular basis. Even nursing home residents can benefit from modest forms of exercise.

An effective exercise program need not be elaborate or expensive. For instance, walking requires a modest investment in shoes and clothing. Dancing and gardening also require little financial outlay.

Poor Environmental Engineering

Policy makers and urban planners should be aware that their work can go a long way in creating an environment that supports physical activity. Examples of good environmental engineering that facilitate physical activity include:

- Well developed and designed sidewalks and bike paths that interconnect to places of interest
- Safe parks that encourage activities of all ages and skill levels

PRESCRIPTION FOR PHYSICAL ACTIVITY

The inaugural *Physical Activity Guidelines for Americans* published in 2008 by the U.S. Department of Health and Human Services represents a big step forward in developing a consensus statement on physical activity for Americans age six and older.[7] The guide is simple to interpret, is comprehensive, and evidence-based.

I recommend that people see their healthcare provider prior to engaging in any physical activity program. Some individuals might need to undergo exercise tolerance testing to determine their ability to tolerate increased cardiovascular demand. Indeed, if you are over age 40, or if you have cardiovascular risk factors, such as diabetes, high cholesterol, and high blood pressure, or a family history of these conditions, you'll need to undergo a comprehensive check-up before embarking on any vigorous exercise program. Be sure to discuss with your healthcare provider your proposed training program to ensure that it's safe to implement and, if safe, how to go about implementing it.

Once cleared to exercise by your healthcare team, you should develop a solid fitness plan that has safety at its core. Your fitness plan should include the following five components: aerobic exercise; muscular strength; muscular endurance; flexibility and balance; and body composition.

The FITT Principle

The American Council on Exercise recommends using the acronym FITT to help remember the elements of your physical activity program. FITT stands for frequency, intensity, timing and type. Let's now examine each piece of a FITT prescription.

Frequency. The American College of Sports Medicine recommends that adults should exercise most days of the week. The American Academy of Pediatrics recommends that children engage in physical activity every day of the week.

Intensity. You can use the ability to hold a conversation to gauge your exercise intensity. Light exercise intensity allows you to carry on a conversation while walking; moderate intensity makes conversation a bit challenging; highly intense exercise makes breathing labored and conversation difficult.

You can calculate your exercise by using your target heart rate. Most healthy people should aim for exercise intensity between 60 percent and 80 percent of their target heart rate. You can calculate your target heart rate using the following formula: 60 percent to 80 percent of 220 minus your age in years. Thus, if you are 50 years old, calculate your target heart rate as follow:

220 minus 50 = 170 multiplied by 0.6 =102 (if you use the 60 percent rate)

or

220 minus 50 = 170 multiplied by 0.8 = 136 (if you use the 80 percent rate)

Thus, if you are 50 years old, your pulse during exertion should be maintained between 102 and 136 beats per minute.

Time. The 2008 *Physical Activity Guidelines for Americans* recommends all adults engage in at least 2½ hours of moderate aerobic physical activity each week, and children engage in at least one hour of physical activity a day.

Type of Exercise. Physical activity need not be complicated or expensive. Choose from menus of both aerobic and anaerobic exercises. Walking is an excellent choice of aerobic exercise because it can be pursued by most people and its relatively low impact protects the lower extremities from injuries. Hiking, gardening, swimming, cycling and jogging are also good outdoor physical activities. Indoor aerobic activities include dancing and using stationary equipment such as the elliptical machine.

I also recommend functional exercises to build core muscle strength that can help prevent falls and help you perform your activities of daily living. A simple way to build core strength is to stand on one leg a few times each day. Start by holding onto the back of a chair and balancing for a count of 20 before switching sides. When you get better, do it without using a chair. You can then do it while washing dishes or brushing your teeth. Closing your eyes provide additional challenge and will further strengthen your core.

Strength training can be fun when using the proper technique. Poor technique can lead to serious injuries, including those involving the neck, arms, back, knees, and ankles. If you are unfamiliar with weight lifting procedures, you should seek help from a fitness instructor. If you have high blood pressure, you should get medical clearance from your doctor.

Yoga is considered the best exercise for achieving flexibility. As I discuss in Chapter 7, this ancient philosophy rooted in Hinduism, emphasizes mind-body connection. Its series of exercise positions also acts upon various joints, including those that are under utilized during the course of a typical day. Yoga also helps tone flaccid and weak muscles. You can take yoga via group fitness classes or do it on your own by viewing yoga DVDs.

Getting Started

An effective and successful exercise program requires careful planning. Ask your doctor and personal trainer to help you select an exercise program and fitness goals. With goals in mind, schedule your exercise sessions like you would schedule other important activities. This will elevate exercise to similar level of importance as going to the hairdresser and ensure compliance. An "exercise buddy" can also provide you with the motivation to stick with your exercise program.

Choose an alternate location and regimen in case inclement weather or other factors preclude exercising. Again, you should start slowly and work your way up. Trying to do too much too soon will likely result in fatigue, burnout, and possibly injury. Start with perhaps a moderately paced walk, and then increase your speed or distance based on your exercise tolerance and rate of improvement.

Go for it!

You won't regret incorporating regular exercise into your life. You'll feel better, look younger, live longer, avoid a long list of preventable diseases, save lots of money, and build a rich social network of friends and acquaintances. Remember, however, while the physiological benefits accrue almost immediately, it might take time for these benefits to become apparent to you. Don't give up after a week if your blood pressure remains unchanged or your self-confidence fails to go through the roof. It will eventually occur—go for it!

IN SUMMARY

- A dubious legacy of the last millennium is that we've developed perfect strategies for maximizing productivity while minimizing physical effort.
- The human body was meant to be moved; fail to use it and you lose it!
- The high price of physical inertia includes: depression, anxiety and excessive stress; impaired cognitive function; overweight and obesity; cardiovascular disease; diabetes; osteoporosis; and cancer.
- There are very few *legitimate* barriers to physical activity but many *perceived* barriers.
- Aerobic exercise (e.g., walking, jogging, swimming, dancing, gardening, and hiking) can be as effective as drugs in lowering mild high blood pressure, high cholesterol and triglycerides, and high blood sugar!
- An effective exercise program need not be expensive or complicated.
- The 2008 *Physical Activity Guidelines for Americans* recommends that all adults engage in at least 2½ hours a week of moderate aerobic physical activity, and children engage in at least one hours of physical activity a day.

Chapter 5

Maintain a Healthy Body Weight

"Overweight and obesity is the second leading cause of death, killing 300,000 people a year. There is not a miracle pill that will lead to weight loss."
—Dr. Richard Carmona
17th Surgeon General of the United States

The statistics pertaining to body weight for Americans are alarming! In 2007, the Centers for Disease Control and Prevention estimated that 66 percent of American adults were overweight or obese. Furthermore, 13 percent of children aged 6 to 11 and 14 percent of adolescents aged 12 to 19 are overweight.

Studies endorsed by numerous health agencies such as the American Heart Association and the American Cancer Society have shown that overweight and obesity cause numerous chronic diseases and shortens life expectancy. Persons who exceed their ideal body weight (see Appendix IV) are at risk for developing type 2 diabetes, high cholesterol, and high blood pressure. As a matter of fact, obese persons (defined as a body mass index of 30 kg/m^2 or higher) are two to six times more likely than their non-obese counterparts to develop hypertension, whether or not the condition runs in the family.

Even a modest increase above one's ideal body weight places excess strain on the heart and blood vessels; it places more pressure on the cardiovascular system to pump blood through the resistance imposed by extra fat tissue. Obesity is associated with hyperinsulinemia, which leads to sodium and water retention and increased blood volume (see Chapter 2). Obese individuals also have higher levels of the hormone adrenaline, which narrows blood vessels and drives up blood pressure (see Chapter 2).

Conversely, achieving a body weight that's healthy for your height is an important anti-aging strategy. An epidemiological study in 2001 showed that higher weight gain correlated with age-related diseases and longevity.[1] Clinically, modest weight loss–even before achieving ideal body weight–can significantly lower blood pressure, blood sugar, triglycerides and cholesterol levels. For example, a 10-pound weight loss can cause a 10 mm Hg and 8 mm Hg reduction in systolic and diastolic blood pressures, respectively.

WHY THE EPIDEMIC OF OVERWEIGHT AND OBESITY?

The reasons for the meteoric rise of overweight and obesity among Americans is the subject of many scientific and clinical debates. Some experts place the blame squarely on the horrific state of our food supply. Others blame our culture of physical inactivity. Yet, others indict excessive stress, poor quality sleep, and other sociocultural factors. No one, however, blames genetics alone for this epidemic.

As I discussed in Chapter 2, weigh gain results from complex biopsychosocial factors that include excessive stress, overeating, under exercising and not getting quality sleep. These factors can independently induce weight gain and together they act synergistically to pile on the pounds!

BARRIER TO ACHIEVING HEALTHY WEIGHT

Well-Worn Excuses

Perhaps the most common reason people fail to lose weight is the list of excuses they astutely craft and honed over a given period of time. As discussed in the previous chapter, some of the more common excuses for not exercising include:

- "I'm too busy."
- "It's dark during the time I can exercise."

- "It's always raining."
- "My feet hurt when I walk."
- "I'm in poor physical shape."
- "I'm too old to exercise."
- "I can't afford to exercise."

These excuses hardly hold water! People almost always find the time to do the things they *perceive* as important. Considering that a good exercise program takes only about 150 minutes each week, everyone's schedule can accommodate a few 30-minute exercise sessions per week. Whether it's less time watching TV or talking on the telephone, *everyone* can find time to exercise. Physical inertia imposes poor musculoskeletal function (as evidenced by pain and windedness) but this can be reversed with an effective physical activity program.

Unhealthy Body Image

A common barrier to achieving proper body weight is an unhealthy body image. We know of eating disorders (e.g., anorexia nervosa and orthorexia nervosa) where sufferers have a distorted body image of being overweight. I think the opposite is also true: overweight people believing that they are underweight. How does this happen? Based on what we know from people with the traditional eating disorders, a distorted body image is born out of rationalization, the self-esteem preserving strategy employed to continue on a desired behavioral path.

Poor Relationship with Food

As discussed in Chapter 2, our attitude about food is an important determinant of our eating habits and, thus, our weight. Surveys reveal that the vast majority of individuals who abuse food do so because of an abnormal relationship with food. Part of the problem is our utter confusion about what to eat, how to eat, when to eat! Michael Pollan, whom I mentioned earlier, largely blames the advent of food science for this unfortunate phenomenon. This new science has spawned a huge database of conflicting results that have created widespread doubt in the minds of the public.

Most of us can't recall the last time we were hungry! We eat, not because of stomach discomfort, but due to a long list of cues such as stress, anxiety, depression, boredom, TV commercials and other automatic triggers. Before you eat, stop and ask yourself whether or not you are really hungry. If you can honestly answer in the affirmative, go ahead and eat. Conversely, if the answer is "no", put away the food and do something else.

Excessive Stress

As we'll discuss in Chapter 7, chronic emotional stress (i.e., distress) can increase one's appetite, facilitate fat storage and cause weight gain. Chronic distress leads to excessive cortisol secretion, which in turn moves fat from various storage sites to visceral storage sites deep in the abdomen.[2] In a study conducted by researchers at Yale University, women with high waist-to-hip ratios (more fat storage in the waist than in the hips) secreted more cortisol under stress than their peers with low waist-to-hip ratios.[3]

PRESCRIPTION FOR A HEALTHY BODY WEIGHT

Overweight and obesity were rare among our ancestors. What's clear is that our fore-parents consumed healthier foods, engaged in more physical activity, and maintained healthy calorie deficit profiles. Our ancestors pursued simpler lives and, as a result, were also less stressed out and less depressed.

In my clinical practice, I recommend a holistic and comprehensive lifestyle modification for most patients seeking to lose weight. I believe that in order to lose weight, most people have to eat healthfully, get appropriate levels of daily physical activity, get quality and adequate quantity of sleep, and manage their stress. However, all of your efforts must be codified in a solid weight-loss plan.

Develop a Written Plan

I recommend you review my discussion of the elements of a Wellness Life Plan in Chapter 1. As with any goal, the starting point for a successful weight loss program is a comprehensive strategic plan. A written plan gives life to your goals and improves your chances for maintaining long-term commitment. Your plan should include: why (your reasons for wanting to lose weight); what (your goal weight); when (timelines); and how (method for losing weight). Your plan should be specific, measurable, achievable, realistic and a have timeline. Before embarking on your weight loss quest, you should discuss your weight loss plan with your healthcare provider and personal trainer.

Health reasons are the best reasons for aspiring to your ideal body weight. Your goal weight must be realistic. Aiming for an unachievable weight is the best way to set yourself up for failure. Like your goal weight, your timelines should be realistic and achievable. A safe weight loss for most people is about 1 to 2 pounds a week (use this guideline to help determine how long it will take to achieve your goal weight). Your healthcare provider can help select the best weight-loss method for you. Generally, most weight-loss methods should include four components, if applicable: nutrition; exercise; sleep schedule; and stress management.

Eat Healthfully

As I discussed in Chapter 2, most overweight and obese persons need to restrict their daily intake of dietary cholesterol and saturated fat, and consume calories commensurate with their body mass index. Obviously, each person is different and consulting a dietitian to obtain a custom-fit diet and personal trainer for an exercise program is appropriate for some. Check with your primary care provider.

Daily Physical Activity

Daily physical activity is an indispensable component of a successful weight-loss plan. As I discussed in Chapter 4, you don't need to run marathons. In fact, you don't need to run at all. The most important elements of a physical activity program are consistency, variety, and familiarity. You should consistently engage in daily physical activity. You should select from a variety of activities to stave off boredom. Finally, you should be familiar with the activity that you select. If your daily physical activity regimen involves a "fun" factor, that's icing on the cake.

Besides walking, you can hike, garden or dance to satisfy your daily physical activity regimen. I also recommend functional exercises to help prevent falls. This type of exercise involves building core muscle strength. One of the simplest ways to strengthen your core is to stand on one leg a few times each day (e.g., while washing dishes or brushing your teeth). Start by holding onto the back of a chair and balancing for a count of 20 before switching sides. When you get better, do it without using a chair. Closing your eyes add an additional challenge and will further improve your core fitness levels.

Get Quality Sleep

As you'll read in Chapter 6, poor quantity and quality sleep correlate with weight gain and, therefore, your weight loss plan must include a sleep schedule that will contribute to a healthy weight. Generally speaking, most adults should get between 7 and 9 hours of sleep each night—even on weekends.

Manage Your Stress

In recent years, scientists have implicated stress as a discrete factor in weight gain (see Chapter 7). Therefore, any weight loss effort must involve the management of excess stress. Distress can zap motivation and commitment and derail physiological mechanisms concerned with weight loss.

HOW TO LOSE FIVE POUNDS IN THE NEXT 30 DAYS

I think it's worth repeating my recommendations from Chapter 2 for losing weight. As a society, we are thoroughly confused about the physiology of weight reduction. The best way to ensure sustained and permanent weight loss is to develop the daily habit of a healthy lifestyle. The following represent a synthesis of healthy ways of living based on current scientific evidence:

- Eat breakfast. After fasting all night, the last thing you want to do is to keep fasting. Skipping breakfast has been shown to slow your metabolism and body's fat-burning capacity.
- Choose from a variety of food groups.
- Eat two healthy snacks at 10:00 am and 2:00 pm. This strategy can help rev up your metabolism and reduce the tendency to overeat at lunch and dinner. Healthy snack choices include a variety of nuts, yogurt, smoothies, fruits and vegetables, popcorn, and trail mixes.
- Eat 10 servings of vegetables and fruits each day. Vegetables and fruits offer unique phytonutrients that support health and wellness. Many of these micronutrients are still being discovered and their roles are yet to be defined.
- Drink enough water to urinate every 3 to 4 hours or so. Water forms the basic biochemical environment for optimal physiological reactions in the body.

- Consume 200 calories at each dinner. This helps you shave off calories from your total intake at the most strategic time of the day (i.e., when you are least active).
- 3 days each week: NO sweets, cakes, pastries, breads. This reduces your weekly burden of simple carbohydrates, a move that can help lower your insulin resistance profile.
- Take a multivitamin/multimineral supplement daily. As I discussed in Chapter 3, this strategy can help fill gaps in your nutrition and lays the foundation for healthy aging by augmenting cell function.
- Sleep 7 to 9 hours each night. Adequate quality and quantity of sleep has global health and wellness benefits and helps your body achieve and maintain healthy a weight (see Chapter 6).
- Review your list of "blessings" at start of each day. This can help mitigate your stress levels, boost self-esteem and prevent over eating. (see Chapter 7).
- Spend 5 minutes of quiet, "me" time every 4 hours. A few minutes of periodic respite has been show to break the cycle of stress that invariably characterizes our day.
- Accumulate at least 10,000 steps on a step counter/pedometer each day. This translates to about three miles of physical activity daily (see Chapter 4).

IN SUMMARY

- A healthy body weight is indispensible to good health, wellness and longevity.

- The reason for our overweight and obesity epidemic is complex and multi-factorial. Factors include: the horrific state of our food supply; our culture of physical inactivity; excessive stress; poor quality sleep; and other sociocultural factors. Genetics alone doesn't explain this epidemic.
- Barriers to achieving a healthy body weight are: crafting well-worn excuses; having an unhealthy body image; having a poor relationship with food; having poor sleeping habits; and harboring excessive stress.
- My prescription for short-term weight loss is to: develop a written plan; eat healthfully; engage in daily physical activity; get quality sleep; and manage your stress.

Chapter 6

Get Quality Sleep

"Early to bed and early to rise, makes a man healthy, wealthy, and wise."
—Benjamin Franklin

The wise admonition of Benjamin Franklin notwithstanding, there's a quiet epidemic thriving in America: from coast to coast, in big cities and small towns, and in neighborhoods of all socioeconomic strata, people are having trouble falling asleep and/or staying asleep. Even if they are able to fall asleep and stay asleep, large numbers of individuals wake up tired and irritable due to poor sleep quality.

The statistics are quite alarming! According to the National Sleep Foundation (NSF), 40 percent of the American population—80 million people—suffer from sleep deprivation.[1] Among the elderly, 50 percent report difficulty falling asleep and/or staying asleep. In a NSF *2005 Sleep in America* poll, 39 percent of respondents admitted to getting less than 7 hours of sleep on weeknights, and 49 percent are so sleep deprived that daytime fatigue interferes with normal daily activities.[1] While Americans today average 6½ hours of sleep each night, Americans in 1960 averaged a full 8 hours of slumber each night. Moreover, an estimated 40 million Americans suffer from one or more of the 70 sleep-related disorders such as sleep apnea, restless leg syndrome, and narcolepsy.

As pervasive as this crisis is, no one seems to notice its existence. In fact, people proudly brag about their ability to function with little sleep; it's the newest macho! Despite this widespread oblivion, sleep deprivation permeates all aspects of our lives: socioeconomic well-being; psychological, emotional, and physical health; and work performance and productivity. Indeed, the direct and indirect cost of insomnia alone is estimated to be $35 billion annually.[1]

Sleep deprivation is one of the most overlooked and under-recognized causes of disease and premature aging. In fact, poor quality and quantity of sleep has been linked to high blood pressure, heart disease, overweight and obesity, and some cancers.[2] In my Wellness practice, I estimate that 90 percent of my patients with chronic diseases experience chronic insomnia. A 2002 poll by the NSF linked poor sleep to the rise in incidence of road rage! Disordered sleep can also exacerbate certain medical conditions such as asthma, arthritis, diabetes, and psoriasis. Additionally, poor depth and length of sleep can result in poor judgment and contribute to auto accidents.

Errors in judgment due to sleep deprivation have been officially linked to tragic industrial accidents, nuclear power plan disasters, and major oil spills. An estimated 37 percent of all vehicle operators admit to having dozed off at the wheel due to a lack of adequate sleep. The National Highway Traffic Safety Administration (NHTSA) estimates that 100,000 crashes resulting in 40,000 nonfatal injuries and 1,500 deaths each year are due to sleep-deprived drivers falling asleep at the wheel.[3]

It should be clearly noted that there are numerous causes of poor sleep, including: sleep apnea; circadian rhythm disorders; neurological conditions, such as restless leg syndrome, narcolepsy, and multiple sclerosis; mental health conditions, such as anxiety and depression; and insomnia. Sleep disorders—even chronic insomnia—are a complex group of conditions that require evaluation by a qualified healthcare practitioner. In this chapter, I'll only address acute and chronic insomnia. I'll explain why sleep is a basic and irreplaceable aspect of our existence and how poor quality and reduced quantity of sleep can contribute to poor health and wellness. I'll also show you how simple strategies can effectively restore the quantity and quality of your sleep.

WHY IS SLEEP SO IMPORTANT?

What exactly is quality sleep? How many hours of sleep does the average person need? What happens in the body when it is not allowed to get the right quality and amount of sleep? Is sleep really that important?

In *The Tempest*, Shakespeare wrote that "We are such stuff....As dreams are made on, and our little life....Is rounded with sleep." Preeminent 19th century American philosopher Ralph Waldo Emerson famously stated that "health is the first muse, and sleep is the condition to produce it." And as noted Russian author and playwright, Anton Pavlovich Chekhov, penned in an 1890 letter to a friend: "I think that it would be less difficult to live eternally than to be deprived of sleep throughout life."

Despite the reverence ancient and contemporary philosophers paid to sleep, its exact biomedical function didn't come into clear focus until the 1950s. Indeed, until the discovery of the rapid eye movement (REM) stage of sleep in 1953, sleep specialists regarded sleep as an inactive, almost insignificant aspect of the human life cycle that resulted from reduced sensory input. A large body of research since the 1960s has shed light on the role of sleep in human health and wellness. That sleep medicine is now a recognizable medical specialty in the United States is testament to the importance of this life phenomenon.

We spend a third of our lives sleeping, and for a good reason: it's as important as eating, exercising, and breathing—necessary for life. According to sleep experts, sleep rejuvenates and retools the immune, nervous, musculoskeletal and endocrine systems of the body.[4] Good quality or restorative sleep equilibrates the entire biochemistry of the body, especially the production of hormones, enzymes, and neurotransmitters—the foundation of optimum health, wellness and life expectancy.

WHAT HAPPENS DURING SLEEP?

Sleep is a complex behavior influenced by circadian rhythms, hormones, enzymes, neurotransmitters, and environmental factors. Contrary to previously held beliefs, sleep is not a passive "down time" where the brain is inactive and the body does nothing. On the contrary, during sleep, the brain and the rest of the body go through an impressive set of measurable neurochemicals and other changes. These changes can be demonstrated on electroencephalography (EEG), a recording of the electrical activity of the brain. These highly specialized events begin during wakefulness and continue during the five cyclic stages of sleep.

The Five Stages of Sleep

The human brain is designed to stay awake for approximately 16 hours without sleep each day. During the last few hours of wakefulness, the brain gradually shuts down, as characterized by a reduction in alertness and cognition. During sleep, the brain enters five distinct patterns of electrical activity that mark the various levels of sleep: stages 1, 2, 3, 4, and rapid eye movement (REM). A good night's sleep involves multiple cycles of these five stages of sleep.

Stage 1 sleep marks the transition from wakefulness to sleep. It is the lightest sleep phase when a person can be easily awakened. Eye movement slows and muscle activity reduces. Stage 2 sleep, which lasts approximately 15 to 20 minutes, can also be classified as a light stage of sleep, and is characterized by a halt in eye movement and slowing of brain waves. In stage 3 sleep, the brain exhibits delta waves, which are very slow electrical activity. In stage 4 sleep, the deepest stage of sleep, the brain enters into a pattern of exclusively delta waves, during which time it's relatively difficult to awaken a person. Finally, in REM sleep, brain waves are low in amplitude and high in frequency (similar to when a person is awake). The eyes move rapidly in all directions, breathing becomes more rapid and shallow, and heart rate and blood pressure increase. Dreaming occurs during the REM phase of sleep.

These sleep phases progress orderly from stage 1 through REM and back to stage 1. A complete sleep cycle from stage 1 to REM sleep averages between 90 and 110 minutes. Thus, a person goes through about 4 sleep cycles during an 8-hour period. The first few sleep cycles usually contain short REM periods and long periods of stages 3 and

4 sleep. Later, REM periods increase and deep sleep periods decrease. Therefore, during an 8-hour sleep period, a person spends a majority of the time in stages 1, 2 and REM sleep.

When the brain fails to traverse the five sleep stages, the body fails to secrete the right amount and types of hormones, neurotransmitters, enzymes and other substances. It can also cause the body to secrete detrimental hormones.

Secretion of Hormones and Neurotransmitters

The brain's ability to go through the various stages of sleep is influenced by neurotransmitters and hormones—brain biochemicals that correlate with the sleep-wake cycle. Scientists are still trying to sort out the precise functions of these biochemicals. The sleep-related hormones and neurotransmitters for which there is solid scientific data include growth hormone, adenosine, melatonin, serotonin, leptin, and grehlin.

Growth Hormone. Also known as somatotropin, growth hormone (GH) is crucial to overall health and wellness: it speeds absorptions of nutrients into cells; helps heal tissues subjected to daily wear-and-tear; and stimulates the bone marrow to produce specialized cells that comprise the immune system. GH also stimulates fat cells to break down triglyceride, suppressing the cells' ability to take up and accumulate circulating lipids. Additionally, GH has a direct effect on protein, fat and carbohydrate metabolism.

GH is produced in the anterior pituitary gland and peaks during sleep stages 3 and 4. Stress, exercise, nutrition and sleep can modulate the production of GH.

Adenosine. One of the most studied brain chemicals is adenosine, which gradually accumulates in the brain during wakefulness but decreases during sleep. Brain and sleep researchers believe that its progressive rise and fall set the stage for sleep quantity and quality. Some people fail to get enough natural light during the day and may under-produce adenosine during the day, resulting in a failure to achieve the levels needed to induce sleep at night.

Melatonin. This hormone, produced in the pineal gland in the brain, is another well-studied sleep-associated brain chemical that appears to be influenced by the circadian clock and darkness. Dubbed "the hormone of darkness," high nighttime levels of melatonin apparently induce sleep in the presence of darkness. Melatonin levels decline at dawn. Some individuals experience "melatonin spillover," persistent production of small amounts of melatonin despite exposure to daylight. Changing time zones and shift work can disrupt circadian rhythms and can negatively influence melatonin production. Melatonin production also wanes as a person ages.

Serotonin. In contrast to melatonin, serotonin (chemical name, 5-hydroxytryptamine or 5-HT) is dubbed "the hormone of wakefulness" because daylight influences its secretion. Produced in an area in the brain stem called the Raphe nuclei, serotonin is believed to play an important role in modulating circadian rhythm and the sleep cycle. Serotonin has also been linked to roles in mood, body temperature, appetite, and physical coordination. Animal studies have shown that blocking the production of serotonin results in sleep disturbances. The precise mechanism of how serotonin affects sleep in humans is currently unclear.

Leptin and Grehlin. These two hormones, found in fat cells, are felt to play a major role in the body's regulation of appetite and insulin/glucose homeostasis. Poor sleep induces a mismatch in leptin and grehlin production. In a landmark study reported in November 2004 at the annual convention of the North American Association for the Study of Obesity, researchers at Columbia University and the Obesity Research Center discovered that the level of leptin (responsible for the feeling of satiety) is decreased with sleep deprivation while grehlin (which inspires hunger pangs) is increased. The study found that, among people age 32 to 59, those who slept four hours or less per night were 73 percent more likely to be obese than those who slept seven to nine hours per night. Apparently, the less you sleep, the more you're likely to be obese.

HEALTH PROBLEMS ASSOCIATED WITH SLEEP DEPRIVATION

Quality sleep is an indispensable component of a healthy lifestyle. As discussed earlier, medical research shows that sleep-deprived individuals are susceptible to poor emotional, mental and physical health. One researcher found that 53 percent of subjects with insomnia reported having two or more health problems compared to only 24 percent of those without insomnia.[5] Chronic sleeplessness can devastate the body's homeostasis and can lead to health problems such as obesity, high blood pressure, immune dysfunction and depression.

People who report less-than-adequate sleep experience generalized musculoskeletal pain and stiffness, headache, and tiredness upon awakening. It is very difficult to get motivated to fully engage in the usual activities of daily living when you start your day in pain and stiffness and fatigued! Poor sleep is also linked to a number of chronic medical conditions such as high blood pressure, heart disease, overweight and obesity, and diabetes.

Altered Immune Function

Experiments done with humans show that sleep deprivation alters immune function, which can lead to infections. Dr. David Dinges and colleagues at the University of Pennsylvania, School of Medicine demonstrated that sleep-deprived subjects experience altered blood levels of white blood cells and natural killer cells, which are specialized immune cells that help the body to fend off germs and prevent disease.[6] Similar results were found among patients with chronic fatigue syndrome (CFS), an arcane condition characterized by persistent, unrelenting fatigue and sleep disturbance. When researchers compared blood samples from a cohort of CFS patients with samples from two control groups, they found a unique pattern of altered cortisol, prolactin, and natural killer cells that accompanied abnormal sleep patterns.[7]

Cognitive Dysfunction

Research scientist, Jan Born, at the University of Lüebeck in Germany says that "during sleep, the brain actively processes information learned during the day." Sleep deprivation, therefore, makes it very difficult to recall learned information. One mechanism might be a surge in stress hormones that can damage the hippocampus, the area in the brain that deals with memory.

Chronic sleep deprivation also leads to a cumulative deficit in attention, comprehension, and judgment. In an elaborate study done jointly at Stanford University and the University of California, Berkeley, researchers found that sleep-restricted rats had a harder time remembering a path through a maze (a task that draws upon memory, attention span and reaction time) compared to their rested counterparts.

As a result of numerous medical errors blamed on lack of sleep, New York State, in 1989, passed sweeping legislation restricting the work hours of medical interns and residents—some of the most sleep-deprived people around—to no more than 80 hours per week over a four-week period. Why was sleep the underlying cause of errors made by these young doctors-in-training? As it turns out, sleep-deprived individuals have shorter attention span, impaired memory, and a longer reaction time—not the kind of cognitive skills you'd want from your doctor!

On the other hand, good quantity and quality sleep can boost the brain's ability to remember recently learned information, according to findings presented at the 59th Annual Scientific Meeting of the American Academy of Neurology in April 2007.[8] Lead researcher, Jeffrey

Ellenbogen of Harvard University Medical School, said that it's "an important message for people in demanding jobs, such as lawyers and doctors, students and senior citizens who already are struggling with mild memory problems." Ellenbogen and his team hired 60 students and had them memorize a list of 20 paired words to test their ability to handle competing information. Sleep-deprived students remembered only 32 percent of the original word pairs while their rested counterparts had 72 percent recall accuracy.

Psychiatric Disorders

Chronic insomnia can lead to depression, anxiety, and substance abuse. In one study, psychiatric disorders accounted for 40 percent of the diagnoses in patients with chronic insomnia.[9] Whether or not the psychiatric disorder caused the insomnia, or vice versa, is debatable. However, another study of nearly 8,000 US adults showed that persons with chronic insomnia at the start of the study were at a 40-fold higher risk of developing subsequent depression within one year, compared with their non-insomniac peers.[10]

As I discussed earlier, during sleep, the human brain goes through five stages of sleep—stage 1 to stage 5 or REM sleep—with each stage lasting a certain length of time. A complete sleep cycle from stage 1 to REM sleep averages between 90 and 110 minutes. In a tantalizing study looking at depression vis-à-vis insomnia, researchers found that subjects who experience early onset of REM sleep were significantly more vulnerable to depression than their peers with a normal sleep profiles.[11] The authors concluded that evaluating sleep pattern might be a way to predict someone's risk for future depression.

High Blood Pressure

Blood pressure is influenced by the body's diurnal clock. Scientists reported in the May 2006 edition of the medical journal *Hypertension* that long-term sleep deprivation increases a person's risk of developing high blood pressure. In a study of 4810 individuals, those who slept less than six hours a night more than doubled their risk for developing elevated blood pressure compared with those who slept more than six hours a night.[12] This study corroborated an earlier study reported in 1996 by Japanese researchers.[13]

Heart Disease

In a study reported at the British Sleep Society in 2007, people who reduced their sleep from 7 hours to 5 hours per night doubled their risk of dying from coronary heart disease.[14] Monitoring 1,255 men with hypertension, Japanese researchers found that those who failed to get at least 7.5 hours of sleep each night were 33 percent more likely to suffer a cardiovascular incident.[15]

Digestive Disorders

Individuals who suffer from circadian-related sleep disruption (e.g., nurses who engage in shift work) report higher rates of digestive problems such as gastroesophageal reflux disease (GERD) and irritable bowel syndrome (IBS). Because the body is meant to eat during the day and sleep at night, working and eating at night is contrary to the normal relationship between the body's internal biorhythms and external stimuli. The dysynchrony thus created induced GERD, IBS, and other functional gastrointestinal conditions.

Overweight and Obesity

As I delineated earlier, sleep-induced hormonal disparity is linked to overweight and obesity. In a study published in the January 10th 2005 issue of *Archives of Internal Medicine*, Dr. Robert Verona and colleagues reported that, among 10001 individuals studied, reduced amounts of sleep directly correlated with increased incidence of overweight and obesity.[16] Many medical and fitness experts believe that the current overweight and obesity trend can partly be blamed on an across-the-board reduction in sleep quantity and quality among Americans.

Pre-diabetes and Diabetes

A lack of sleep affects the hormones that regulate blood sugar (glucose) and appetite. When sleep expert Eva van Cauter of the University of Chicago immunized sleep-deprived students with the flu vaccine, their immune systems failed to produce the predictable number of antibodies, but they produced high levels of cortisol, a hormone associated with stress, weight gain, and pre-diabetes.[17] The subjects also increased their caloric intake by 1000 calories and their blood sugars rose to pre-diabetic levels.

In another small experiment at the University of Chicago, young healthy volunteers between the ages of 20 and 31 showed an inability to regulate their blood sugars when noise disrupted their stage 5 sleep. A co-researcher in this study, Dr. Eva Van Couter, said "these results suggest that strategies to improve sleep quality, as well as quantity, may help to prevent or delay the onset of type 2 diabetes in populations at risk."

HOW MUCH SLEEP DO YOU NEED?

How much sleep do you need each night and what can you do to get the right quantity and quality of sleep? Do you need to get all of your sleep at one time or can you sleep multiple, shorter durations? The amount of sleep necessary is fairly individualized but most experts agree that everyone fall within a range.

Age is the primary determinant of the amount of sleep an individual requires. Newborns require 16 to 20 hours of sleep each day. By age two, children need only 9 to 12 hours of sleep. Teenagers require about 9 to 10 hours of sleep while their middle-age counterparts can get away with 7 to 9 hours of sleep. Older adults require between 7 and 8 hours of uninterrupted sleep each night, according to sleep experts at the National Sleep Foundation.[1] Obviously, there are individual variations with some people requiring more or less than average hours of sleep. However, most authorities recommend that all adults get at least 7 hours of sleep each night. This recommendation also applies to the elderly who often *get* less sleep as they age (due to chronic pain and other health issues) but *need* at least 7 hours.

In term of whether you need to sleep for 7 hours straight or accumulate several short duration of sleep in a 24-hour period (polyphasic sleep), is debatable. Proponents for polyphasic sleep point to astronauts and military personnel who do well with this sleep strategy. Famous polyphasic sleepers include Leonardo De Vince and Thomas Edison—these individuals were hugely successful in their fields of endeavor despite polyphasic sleeping patterns.

Opponents to this strategy point to the paucity of time spent in REM sleep, the stage of sleep when, some scientists believe, the brain and other organs undergo most rejuvenation and retooling. Most medical authorities don't prescribe to routine polyphasic sleep and recommend that we get our 7 to 9 hours of sleep all at one stretch. Additionally, sleeping in on weekends in an attempt to make up for lost sleep during the week is not recommended as it will throw off your biological clock in a way that can affect your weekday sleep.

PRESCRIPTION FOR RESTFUL SLEEP

What does it take to get a restorative night of slumber? My first recommendation for anyone with sleep difficulty is to first see his or her healthcare provider. Even garden variety insomnia should not be left to self-diagnosis. My prescription for a good night's sleep pertains to insomniacs without any identifiable medical cause such as cancer or psychiatric problems. Obviously, the treatment for secondary insomnia—that which is caused by an identifiable medical condition—is directed at the underlying cause and should be evaluated and managed by a physician or other qualified healthcare provider.

How important is sleep to you? In your mind, is it as basic as eating and breathing? Fundamental to any pro-active efforts to achieve quality sleep is the priority assigned to the act of sleeping. If you think that sleep gets in the way of your other activities, you'll effectively put it at the bottom of your "to do" list. On the other hand, if you consider sleep as important to your very existence as good nutrition, you'll nurture it and create all the conditions needed to ensure quality sleep. Therefore, the first order of business is to make sleep a priority in your life.

There are evidence-based factors that can help the vast majority of people get a good night's sleep. Table 6-1 lists the factors that can negatively impact the quality and quantity of sleep. Stimulants such as caffeine; physical, emotional and social conflicts; circadian sleep disorders such as jet lag; and certain medicines and herbs can get in the way of a good night's sleep. These factors can disrupt the body's circadian rhythm and the pineal gland's production of melatonin and serotonin. Clearly, the more than eighty primary sleep disorders such as narcolepsy, restless leg syndrome, obstructive sleep apnea, and sleepwalking are not amenable to self-care and should always be treated by a physician or other qualified health practitioner.

Table 6-1
Factors That Can Negatively Impact Sleep

- Circadian sleep disorders
    - Jet lag
    - Shift work
- Chronic pain
- Stimulants
    - Caffeine
    - Tobacco products
- Toxic emotions
    - Anger
    - Fear
    - Anxiety
- Sleep apnea
- Narcolepsy
- Restless leg syndrome
- Parasomnias
    - Arousal disorder
    - Sleep-wake transition disorder
    - REM sleep disorder

Because the human body is meant to be in synchrony with the cycles of nature, the sleep-wake cycle is designed to mirror daytime-nighttime cycle. Thus, the best time to go sleep is between 10:00 p.m. and 6:00 am. A number of other nighttime strategies (see Table 6-2) can help prepare your brain for sleep and relieve daytime fatigue.

Table 6-2
Prescription for a Good Night's Sleep

- Avoid large evening meals
- Avoid chemical and physical stimulants
- Stay away from sleeping pills and alcohol
- Invest in a good mattress and pillow
- Create good pre-sleep rituals
- Fix the underlying problem(s) of insomnia
- Control chronic pain
- Treat circadian sleep disorders
- Consider natural therapeutics
    - 5-hydroxytryptophane (5-HTP, 5-HT or HTP)
    - Valerian root
    - Melatonin

Avoid Large Evening Meals

The size of your evening meal can impact your sleep. A large meal, especially if consumed within four hours of bedtime, can produce abdominal fullness and heartburn that can disrupt your sleep. Drinking a warm cup of milk with nutmeg and honey can facilitate relaxation. Other good choices include chamomile or valerian root tea.

On the flip side of eating a large meal before bedtime is going to bed hungry. Hunger pangs can be just as distracting and stimulating to the brain as caffeine and nicotine. Similarly, hypoglycemia (low blood sugar) can impair quality sleep.

Since there's a four-hour window between the evening meal and bedtime, you should eat a small, low-glycemic index snack containing protein, about an hour or two before bedtime. Nuts, low-fat yogurt, and turkey strips are good choices for an evening snack. Table 6-3 lists some suggestions for pre-bedtime snacks.

Table 6-3
Top 10 Bedtime Snacks

- Turkey
- Low-fat string cheese
- Almonds
- Wall nuts
- Bananas
- Whole-wheat bread
- Warm milk
- Yogurt
- Chamomile tea
- Peanut butter

Avoid Chemical, Emotional and Physical Stimulants

Refrain from consuming stimulants such as caffeine, tobacco products, and refined sugars for at least four hours before bedtime. Caffeine speeds up the heart, raises blood pressure and prevents the brain from slowing down. Tobacco is a potent stimulant that has the same effects on the body as caffeine. If you smoke cigarettes or use smokeless tobacco, you should quit as soon as possible.

Refined carbohydrates raise blood sugar and insulin levels. Later, when blood sugar level drops, the resulting low blood sugar will affect brain function and wake you up. Toxic emotions (e.g., anger and anxiety) and intense mental stress seem to magnify in the still of the night and can impair sleep. Whatever you do, don't agonize over falling asleep; the resulting anxiety can prevent you from sleeping.

Physical activities can also act as a stimulant and should be avoided starting four hours before bedtime. It is true that some people sleep well despite physical exertion close to bedtime, but if you find that exertion disrupts your sleep cycle, I recommend that you exercise early in the day.

Some prescription and over-the-counter medicines and nutritional supplements (see Tables 6-4 and 6-5) can act as stimulants. It is wise to review your list of medications and supplements with your health practitioner to see if they might be causing undue stimulation that can interfere with your sleep. You might be able to take your medication or supplement a different time of day without having to change medication or supplement.

Table 6-4
Drugs That Can Affect Sleep

- Alcohol
- Caffeine
- Pseudoephedrine
- Lithium
- Propranolol
- Theophylline
- Levodopa

Table 6-5
Herbs and Dietary Supplements That Can Affect Sleep

- Yerba mate
- Guarana
- Ginseng
- Capsaicin
- Bitter Orange
- Kola nut
- Green tea
- All energy drinks

Stay Away From Sleeping Pills and Alcohol

Sleeping aids—especially when consumed over a long period of time—can mask the underlying problem while providing a false sense of security. Some sleeping pills can be addictive. If you have to have a sleeping aid, ask your doctor about using a natural sleep-aid product (see discussion below entitled "If all Else Fails"). Only your doctor can help you make this decision.

Alcohol can create a sense of relaxation and help you fall asleep. However, this effect is only short-lived as alcohol can cause blood sugar swings. Alcohol products can also preclude the brain from traversing the various stages of sleep, specifically interfering with REM sleep.

Invest in a Good Mattress and Pillow

Fundamental to restful sleep is a comfortable sleeping surface. If your mattress is too small, too soft or too hard, and doesn't support your back, your sleep will be restless and you'll wake up tired, irritable and stiff. An incompatible mattress can cause you to toss and turn and impede your brain from traversing the five stages of sleep.

Like a good mattress, having the right pillow can help prevent unnecessary tossing and turning, and neck and shoulder soreness in the morning. A good pillow supports your neck at the angle that's comfortable for you. It should spring back into shape when folded in half. If you have neck or back pain, consider buying a cervical pillow that supports your neck without too much flexion (forward bending). Your chiropractor can provide you with guidance in this regard.

Create Good Pre-sleep Rituals

A good night's sleep requires adequate preparation and the right ambiance. Most adults can achieve good quality sleep if they practice pre-sleep rituals and go to bed and wake up at the same time. Table 6-6 lists suggestions for good pre-sleep rituals.

Table 6-6
Good Pre-sleep rituals

- 4 hours before bedtime
    - Last modest-size meal
    - No caffeine, tobacco or other stimulants
    - No alcohol (interfere with REM sleep)
- 2 hours before bedtime
    - Light protein snack
    - No toxic emotions
    - Warm shower
    - No TV
    - Comfortable temperature
- 1 hour before bedtime
    - Light reading
    - Dimly lit bedroom
    - White noise
    - Remove background noise (ticking clocks)
    - Positive affirmations
- Go to bed at the same time
    - By 10—11 pm

Good pre-sleep rituals include a warm bath, light reading, soft music, prayer, meditation and positive affirmations—whatever works for you—for about 30 minutes before bedtime. A warm bath can help relax the body and slow down a racing mind. It might help to place a few drops of a calming aromatherapy essential oil such as lavender, vanilla or sandalwood in your bath water. You can also burn a candle and listen to soothing music.

Reading can quiet an agitated mind and facilitate quality sleep. Your choice of reading material is very important. For example, reading suspense novels or violent materials may over excite the brain and impede all sleep efforts. Carefully select your pre-sleep reading materials from a list of "soft" topics such as inspirational literature that can help you to wind down and relax.

The temperature and humidity in your bedroom should be comfortable. Use a dehumidifier, heater, or air conditioner to create the ambient temperature that's ideal for you. The amount of clothing you wear can contribute to overheating or cause you to feel too cold. Cold feet can negate all pro-sleep strategies—you should, therefore, wear socks to bed.

The area of the brain that regulates circadian cycles is very sensitive to darkness and light. Darkness is one of the most potent influences for shifting from wakefulness to sleepfulness. An hour before going to bed, dim your room light to the lowest practical level. If you choose to have a light in your bedroom all night, select a soft light that can be dimmed, as needed. Use curtains and shades to block out street lights and other sources of external light.

White noise or nature sounds, such as the sound of forest or ocean, can help relax and prepare the body for sleep. Conversely, watching television, playing video games and working on a computer provide excessive visual and auditory input that can over stimulate the brain. Remove unneeded background noises from your bedroom such as a ticking wall clock. Use a clock radio instead of a battery operated clock, which often produce sleep-disrupting noise.

Consider journaling as a way to dump intrusive thoughts and concerns and quiet the mind. A few minutes of writing down your feelings can help set the stage for falling asleep and staying asleep.

If, despite a good pre-sleep ritual, you are unable to fall asleep after 20 minutes in bed, get up and go to another dimly-lit room and engage in light activities such as reading or positive affirmations. Return to bed only when drowsy.

Fix the Underlying Problem(s) of Insomnia

Insomnia is not a primary disorder; it is usually secondary to another health problem. Therefore, the only way to meaningfully address insomnia is to identify and eliminate its underlying cause(s). People who chronically experience insomnia can point to emotional stress, blood sugar disturbances, heartburn, premenstrual syndrome, medication use, late-night eating, or other factors as the basis for their sleep disorder. Many of my patients report chronic emotional stress that intensifies as they attempt to unwind by reviewing the events in their day, and this causes them to engage in emotional eating. Both emotional stress and a full stomach can combine to preclude a good night's sleep.

If toxic emotions are the culprit, get help from a trained psychotherapist. There are a litany of effective remedies for chronic heartburn and GERD. Talk with your doctor about ways to mitigate your condition.

A common sleep retardant among women is perimenopausal and postmenopausal drop in estrogen levels. The hot flashes and night sweats that characterize this transitional period of life can severely disrupt the quality and quantity of a woman's sleep. There are many effective approaches to managing these symptoms. Your women's healthcare practitioner can help you chart a natural hormonal replacement course.

Control Chronic Pain

If you have chronic pain, work with your doctor to achieve good pain management via the many options available. As a traditional naturopathic doctor, I believe it's best to get to the root cause of pain rather than just treating the symptoms.

Recent breakthrough studies at the University of Michigan show that chronic pain impulses register as an active phenomenon in the brain.[18] Using a specialized type of imaging positron emission tomography, researchers were able to demonstrate changes in brain chemistry that were directly induced by pain. The science now shows that pain prevents the brain from throttling back and relaxing enough to allow for a good night's slumber.

In a study of patients with low back pain, 30 minutes of massage therapy twice weekly for five weeks provided impressive pain relief by boosting serotonin levels.[19] The omega-3 fatty acids, found in fatty fish like salmon and mackerel, have been shown to reduce inflammation and chronic pain. In a study conducted by Dr. Wadie Najim and colleagues at the University of California-Irvine, Sam-e was as effective as Celebrex in reducing arthritis pain.[20]

Treat Circadian Sleep Disorders

The human body operates on a diurnal pattern: External light and darkness influences our internal biological apparatus that control wakefulness and sleepiness. It is, therefore, normal to experience insomnia and other sleep difficulty when changing time zones and when engaged in shift work. Even annual changes in daylight-savings time can prove challenging for some people.

Requiring the body to resynchronize to a new sleep-wake cycle—even a one-hour difference—involves a complex biological adjustment that can take days to achieve. When traveling, try to synchronize your sleep to the time zone to which you are traveling. For example, in a hotel, use a penlight instead of overhead lights if you use the bathroom in the middle of the night in order to avoid disturbing the body's circadian clock. Another strategy is to use the thermostat to keep the temperature at optimal levels. A 30- to 60-minute nap during the day might help make up for loss of sleep during the night, but try not to nap too close to bedtime.

If, despite natural sleep strategies, you are having a hard time adjusting to changes in your circadian rhythm, speak with your healthcare practitioner about medications or supplements that you can use on a temporary basis. Natural products are rapidly becoming the sleep aid of choice for many Americans. I'll discuss these products and others in the next section of this chapter.

WHEN ALL ELSE FAILS

Despite their best efforts, some people need help to sleep. For example, people suffering with fibromyalgia, an enigmatic disease that affects nearly 10 million Americans, have long-term difficulty with quality and quantity of sleep. Some of these individuals can benefit from taking a sleep aid at bedtime. Are pharmaceutical sleeping pills the answer? Sedative-hypnotics, the class of drugs under which sleeping pills fall, have been associated with bizarre side effects. In recent years, as more and more people take these drugs, a large number of reports describe dangerous side effects. Clearly, when needed, these agents should be prescribed and closely monitored by a qualified healthcare professional.

Natural sleep aids include 5-hydroxytryptophane (also referred to as 5-HTP, 5-HT or HTP), valerian root, melatonin, *Schisandra chinensis*, *Ziziphus spinosa*, and *Polygala tenuifolia*. Compared with pharmaceutical agents, these natural products impose fewer side effects and are usually nonaddictive.

5-hydroxytryptophane (5HTP)

The amino acid, 5-hydroxytryptophane (5-HTP), is derived from the seeds of *Griffonia Simplicofolia*, a plant native to West and Central Africa. It is very effective at smoothing out rough spots in the sleep cycle.[21] This product converts in the brain into serotonin, an important brain chemical that regulates mood, appetite and sleep. The recommended dose of 5-HTP is 50—100 mg taken on an empty stomach one hour before bedtime. Side effects include nausea, vomiting and stomach cramps. Don't take 5-HTP with other supplements or drugs that alter serotonin levels such as Sam-e and fluoxitine. How long you should take 5-HTP is questionable. Check with your healthcare provider for his or her recommendation.

Valerian Root

Used for thousands of years as a sedative herb, valerian root is also an effective sleep aid for some people. Derived from a plant native to both North America and Europe, valerian root helps regulate the brain chemical gama-aminobutryic acid (GABA), which slows brain excitation. There are wide variations in consistency of various commercially available valerian products, so select your supplement from a reputable company. The recommended dose of valerian root is 300—400 mg taken on an empty stomach one hour before bedtime. It might take a few days to realize the full effects of the herb. Side effects include a feeling of wooziness in the morning and headache.

Melatonin

As I discussed earlier, melatonin is produced in the body in a diurnal pattern to induce sleep. Tart red cherries are a natural source of melatonin. Recommended dose of supplemental melatonin is between 0.3 and 2.5 mg before bedtime. Side effects include abdominal cramping, mild irritability and increased dreams, including vivid dreams. Because melatonin can narrow blood vessels, individuals with blood vessel disorders should not take this supplement. Pregnant women should not take melatonin.

Other Sleep Aids

Traditional Chinese Medicine (TCM) gives us three effective sleep aids: *Schisandra chinensis*, *Ziziphus spinosa*, and *Polygala tenuifolia*. *Schisandra chinensis*, *Schisandra* is a fruit extract that has been used for centuries as a vital adaptogen—an agent used to help the body adapt to emotional stress. *Ziziphus spinosa* is a popular TCM herb used to relax and calm the soul. Finally, *Polygala tenuifolia* is an herb used to enhance mental faculties and promote sound sleep. Check with a TCM-trained herbalist for recommendations on how to use these products.

IN SUMMARY

- Sleep disturbance is at epidemic proportions among Americans, affecting an estimated 40 percent of the population.
- Sleep length and breadth are as important as any other physiological function such as breathing and eating.
- Health problems linked to poor sleep include overweight and obesity, high blood pressure, and depression.
- There are five distinct stages of sleep, each characterized by unique brain-wave patterns and muscle tension.
- Adults require 7 to 9 hours of uninterrupted sleep every night.
- Strategies for ensuring a good night's sleep include creating the right sleep environment; treating issues causing insomnia; staying away from stimulant drugs and supplements; avoiding sleeping pills and alcohol; managing chronic pain; treating circadian sleep disorders; and talking with your healthcare provider about natural therapies, as a last resort.
- Natural sleep aids include 5-hydroxytryptophane (also referred to as 5-HTP, 5-HT or HTP), valerian root, melatonin, *Schisandra chinensis*, *Ziziphus spinosa*, and *Polygala tenuifolia*.

Chapter 7

Manage your Stress

"To avoid sickness eat less; to prolong life worry less."
—Chu Hui Weng

Like oxygen, emotional stress is ubiquitous! From minor everyday annoyances to life-altering loses, modern life is fraught with stressors. Most people can relate to unpleasant events, uncompromising demands, escalating expectations, and excessive noise as germane to their daily lives. Indeed, experts in behavioral medicine will tell you that stress is an intrinsic and inseparable part of life—stress is life, life is stress!

Is stress beneficial or detrimental to overall health and aging? What are the short-term benefits of a racing heart and tense muscles? What are the long-term health consequences of excessive demand and unrealistic expectations? In this chapter, I'll discuss the various dimensions of psychological stress: what it is and isn't; what happens in the body during stress; the health problems it imposes; and offer a practical recipe for managing daily stress.

WHAT IS STRESS?

Everyone knows what stress is but there is hardly consensus about its definition. Psychologists have their definition for stress. Business consultants have theirs. Medical professionals also define stress in their own way. Who has the right definition? Is it possible to achieve a unified definition for this ambiguous emotional experience?

Stress is a very personal experience. An event that is non-stressful for one person can be severely stressful (i.e., distressful) for another. The largely subjective nature of this life experience precludes a single definition. However, despite a lack of consensus, most behavioral specialists agree that stress is a *perceived* threat—real or imagined—to one's physical or mental well-being. The perception is grounded in the belief that a given demand has outstripped the resources one can bring to bear. More fundamentally, the genesis of a person's perception is deeply rooted in his or her genetic endowment, personal experiences, and environmental influences.

Is stress positive or negative or, can it be both negative and positive? We invariably speak of stress with disdain and scorn. Yet, most authorities agree that, while excessive stress can be detrimental, a stress-free life also can be deleterious to our growth, development and well-being. Up to a point, stress serves to help us build "psychological muscles" that arm us with the ability to react to life's many challenges. Each individual has an optimal positive stress level, dubbed *eustress*—the impetus for creativity and motivation to effectively deal with everyday events. Eustress improves our concentration, focus, and cognitive ability.

On the other hand, excessive stress is overwhelming and serves as *distress*. This is the point at which biochemical changes in the body exact a huge physical, emotional and spiritual toll. Indeed, the mind-body interplay related to stress is the subject of numerous medical studies, the results of which are starting to illuminate the complex biopsychosocial response to excessive stress.

WHAT HAPPENS DURING EXCESSIVE STRESS?

From time to time, most of us suffer from some degree of distress. Whether or not stress is perceived as distress depends mostly on its intensity, its duration, and the person's ability to cope.

Psychologists characterize our reaction to stress as the "fight-or-flight" response, which is traceable to our primordial existence, a time when we had to physically respond to menacing wild animals and other life-threatening events. Biologically speaking, the stress response involves a complex interplay between the nervous system and a series of hormones (called catecholamines) that prepare us to deal *physically* with a perceived *physical* threat. All of this takes place in the "stress circuit," technically referred to as the hypothalmus-pituitary-adrenal (HPA) axis.

Catecholamines (namely, dopamine, norepinephrine and epinephrine) secretion cause numerous physiological changes in the body, including rapid heartbeat, increased blood pressure, rapid and shallow breathing, and increased clotting potential of the blood. Cortisol, a steroid hormone secreted into the blood from the adrenal glands, causes the release of free fatty acids (i.e., triglycerides) into the blood, depression of brain cell activity, breakdown of tissues, and suppression of the immune system.

During pre-historic times, when wild animals threatened our very existence, it was imperative for humans to have a ready supply of catecholamines to provide the extra energy and physical skills needed to stay and fight or to run away. Such responses were short lived—you either fought off the ensuing prey or died trying to defend yourself. Today, most of our threat are not physical in nature but *emotionally* derived from the frenetic pace and challenges imposed by modern living. The demands of modern life—work, family, relationships, etc—exact a high toll in terms of toxic emotions such as anxiety, anger, and depression. Common modern-day acute stressors include deadlines, work overload, loud noise, loss of prestige or status, physical illness, and threats to self-esteem. Chronic stressors include sleep deprivation, chronic pain, divorce, and social isolation.

Chronic distress (i.e., an overactive HPA axis) results in prolonged release of cortisol which, in addition to suppressing the immune system and other dysfunction, stimulates the appetite and contributes to fat storage and weight gain.[1] In addition, a chronically distressed individual commonly develops chronic, low levels of anger, anxiety and depression. Over time, these toxic emotions affect the way the person feels, thinks, and behaves. As a result, the individual's concentration wanes, thinking clouds, and he makes poor decisions. Under these circumstances, most people indulge in destructive behaviors (e.g., excessive use of food, drugs, and alcohol). Ultimately, health problems ensue.

HEALTH PROBLEMS ASSOCIATED WITH STRESS

Not only is stress difficult to define; it's hard to measure objectively, which is why it's difficult to connect it to the development of diseases. Nevertheless, the physical and emotional effects of persistent and unremitting distress are readily apparent. Table 7-1 lists the warning symptoms of excessive psychological stress.

As I discussed earlier, during prolonged stress, the heart races, breathing quickens, the mind races, and thinking blurs. What are the negative health effects of these physiological responses we call stress? A large body of research in the past few decades has catalogued a long list of health conditions linked to chronic emotional stress. The American Psychological Association estimates that 75 percent to 90 percent of all visits to a physician are linked to stress.[2] These conditions include accelerated aging, skin disorders, sleep disturbances, headache, depression, heart disease, high blood pressure, gastrointestinal diseases, and overweight and obesity. Additionally, excessive stress has been shown to exacerbate chronic medical conditions such as asthma, diabetes, and arthritis.

Table 7-1
Warning Symptoms of Excessive Stress

Cognitive
- Poor memory
- Clouded thinking
- Poor decision making

Emotional
- Anger
- Feeling overwhelmed
- Moodiness
- Anxiety
- Depression

Behavioral
- Excessive use of alcohol
- Overeating
- Tobacco use
- Teeth grinding during sleep

Physical
- Insomnia
- Dizziness
- Headaches
- Chest pain
- Palpitation
- Indigestion
- Muscle stiffness

Accelerated Aging

Distress is one of the most age-accelerating influences there is, perhaps on the same level as smoking. Excessive stress increases the level of free radicals, hastens protein breakdown, suppresses the immune system, and ages DNA—all factors that cause the body to age faster than normal.

Skin Problems

Most skin doctors agree that emotional stress can exacerbate various skin disorders. People who suffer from eczema, psoriasis, dandruff, herpes, hives and acne, report flares of their condition during times of excessive stress. Medical studies show a positive correlation between the number of flare-ups of genital herpes rash and levels of stress.[3] On the other hand, stress management techniques such as meditation and yoga effectively reduce the number of herpes outbreaks. Surveys of acne suffers reveal a strong connection between emotional distress and worsening of acne.[4]

Sleep Disturbances

What's the connection between excessive stress—distress—and sleep disturbance? As you learned in Chapter 6, sleep occurs in the brain, and trying to fall asleep or stay asleep with a "loud" brain is nearly impossible. Excess stress alters brain function, impairing one's ability to fall asleep and stay asleep. In fact, the epidemic of distress among Americans mirrors the epidemic of sleep disturbances.

Headache

There is no official classification of "stress headache" but there ought to be! Nevertheless, tension-type headache—the most common type of headache—has deep roots in excessive stress. Stress is also a common trigger for migraine headaches.

Depression

Excessive cortisol secretion interferes with the production and action of brain neurotransmitters, mainly dopamine and serotonin. This biochemical pattern is detected in depressed individuals. Invariably, the root causes are daily stressors such as family conflict, financial difficulties and loss of job.

Thyroid Dysfunction

Endocrinologists, doctors who treat disorders such as those of the thyroid gland, report that stress-induced cortisol can affect the conversion of thyroid hormone from its inactive to active form. Even though the thyroid gland makes adequate amounts of thyroid hormone, these compounds never get to their target organs.

Heart Disease

Heart disease is probably the best-known health condition associated with excessive emotional stress. Numerous studies have demonstrated that people with Type A personalities—i.e., driven, competitive, impatient and aggressive—experience more heart attacks than their Type B peers.[5] Not surprising, since Type A persons show a high prevalence of elevated cholesterol, triglycerides, blood pressure, insulin, and catecholamines.

High Blood Pressure

A large body of studies reveals a connection between chronic stress and high blood pressure (also called hypertension). One prominent study revealed that emotional stress on the job apparently influences the secretion of norepinephrine and epinephrine, which stimulate the nervous system and raise blood pressure.

Scientists at the University of California, School of Medicine found that mice living in crowded cages developed hypertension, while those living in spacious environments did not. Social scientists speculate that the stress of poverty, poor living conditions, and low socioeconomic and educational status might partly explain the high prevalence of hypertension among African Americans.

Gastrointestinal Diseases

The brain and the gastrointestinal system are interrelated and mediated by the same hormones. Not surprisingly, excessive emotional stress changes intestinal motility and produces excessive stomach acid. Indeed, acute life-threatening stress such as post-traumatic stress disorder has been linked to the development of functional gastrointestinal disorders such as irritable bowel syndrome.[6]

Even though most stomach and duodenal ulcers have been linked to either an infection with the *Helicobacter Pylori* bacteria or the use of non-steroidal anti-inflammatory drugs, psychological stress is still regarded as a contributing factor in the majority of cases of peptic ulcers.[7]

Overweight and Obesity

As I discussed earlier, researchers have linked chronic emotional stress to increased appetite, fat storage and weight gain. Chronic distress leads to excessive cortisol secretion, which in turn moves fat from various storage sites to visceral storage sites deep in the abdomen.[8] In a study conducted by researchers at Yale University, women with high waist-to-hip ratios (more fat storage in the waist than in the hips) secreted more cortisol under stress than their peers with low waist-to-hip ratios.[9]

BREAKING THE STRESS CYCLE

If stress is intimately connected to our perception of an event, then a good starting point for managing stress is to manage our perception of that event. How do you implement such cognitive restructuring? How do you think differently about a "stressful" event, interaction, or other encounter?

Changing poor thinking takes a lot of work. Stress-relieving maneuvers are easily learned and practiced. These techniques include biofeedback, yoga, progressive muscle relaxation, and visualization. The physical activity program we previously discussed is also an excellent stress management tool. It is also important to get adequate amounts of sleep. You'll also find that hot baths, massage (including self-massage), and relaxing music have calming effects, and may be employed as stress management strategies.

Identify Your Stressors

The first step in managing your stress is to identify *your* stressors by writing down all events and factors that are the sources of your angst. Since stress is a personal experience, your list of stressors will likely be different from someone else exposed to your environment.

The most common causes of stress are financial problems, job dissatisfaction, relationship discord, and health problems. How do you identify *your* stressors? What should you write down? In some cases, it might not be easy to determine what bothers you. However, your stress warning symptoms (see Table 7-1) will help you associate events that trigger a stressful reaction. For example, think of the events that make you angry and anxious, such as slow moving traffic. In this case, traffic jams represent one of your stressors. Do this exercise until you've identified all of your stressors.

Develop Healthy Ways of Thinking

Poor thinking is the breathing ground for negative cognitive processing that cultivates anger, anxiety, resentment, and other toxic emotions.

Knowing how you think is just as important as knowing what are your life stressors. Einstein said that you can't solve a problem with the same head that created the problem. If poor thinking is the source of skewed perception, you have to learn ways to think positively.

Our thinking patterns are part learned behavior, part genetics. Researchers at Yale University identified a mutated gene that codes for rumination, the cognitive process that can cultivate negative thinking. But, genetic endowment doesn't mean destiny: you can effectively learn to overcome this genetically-driven challenge, if present. How do you do this? I recommend that you make a list of things that are right with your life and a second list of things that are wrong with your life. The act of writing down your past experiences gives life to both good and bad experiences and invariably will show you that things are not as bad as your mind will lead you to believe—the list of good things is invariably longer than the list of bad things.

Learning to think positively can be difficult for some people but you can start putting a positive spin on small events and experiences. During heavy traffic, for example, accept the facts that during rush hour, there will be dense traffic. Ensure you are breathing deeply, which relieves physical tension (see "Practice Relaxation Techniques" below). Finally, spend the down time rehearsing for an important meeting later in the day.

Practice Mindfulness

Common causes of stress are wandering and uncontrollable thoughts that are firmly planted in the past and the future. Mindfulness is the act of focusing the mind exclusively on the here and now. Championed by mind-body pioneer, Dr. Herbert Benson, of Harvard Medical School, mindfulness helps to slow the mind and focus on one mental activity at a time.

Mastering mindfulness requires lots of practice. Start by deeply experiencing your immediate environment and what's going on around you. Stop and smell the rose. Savor the chirping of birds. Listen to the water flow in the nearby river.

Next, try practicing the art of gratitude—being thankful for your many blessings. In Japan, where I live, people are ever aware and thankful for the things they *do* have. In contrast, in the West, people constantly think of the things they *don't* have. Get in the habit of being thankful for your many accomplishments, relationships, good health, etc—all the things that you *do* have.

Establish Boundaries Between Various Aspects of Your Life

In our 24/7 lifestyle, the various functional areas of our lives seems to converge into one big ill-defined demand. With the advent of advanced electronic media—e-mail, laptop computers, cell phones, and BlackBerries—we can communicate 24 hours a day with family, friends and co-workers, making it difficult to separate our personal life from our work life. This lack of clear boundaries between responsibilities can prove dizzying and can diminish our functional efficacy. As a result, we are doing office work while juggling family responsibility and fighting to get quiet time for ourselves while exercising.

Time Allocation. A healthy life plan is to develop well-defined compartments in your life—and stick to them! Work time is from 8 am to 5 pm; family time, from 6 pm to 9 pm; personal time, between 9 pm and bedtime; etc. Resolve to never check work-related e-mail from home, and vice versa. You might want to screen calls coming to your cell phone and answer business-related calls only during business hours. These strategies will help ensure that you leave work-associated stress at work and not entertain them while you interact with your family.

What happens to those of you who don't have the resources to manage the boundaries you set for yourself? What do you do if your boss, co-workers, friends or relatives fail to respect the boundaries that you set for your life? Like any change in life, it'll take time to implement. You might have to manage a single boundary at a time. For example, you can start with your personal life boundaries because you are in better control of them. For your work-related boundaries, inform your co-workers of your intention to establish various boundaries and enlist their help to maintain them.

Learn to Say No! Another strategy for establishing limits in your life is to learn to say "NO" when your demands outstrip your resources. Invariably, people who can't say "no" when it's appropriate to do so are life-long people pleasers. Entering into new commitments when you don't have the resources to do so is done out of a strong desire to please others. Eventually, you can't keep up with your many commitments and you'll let people down—and this can be very stressful!

But there's a way to break this viscous cycle. The first thing to do is to realize that saying "no" is not selfish; it's beneficial to your other commitments. An inevitable consequence of having too much on your plate is failure to effectively meet *any* of your commitments. Develop ways to politely—but firmly—decline requests for your time: "Sorry, my dance card is full at this time; I'll consider your request in the near future." So, let go of your guilt of having to say "no!"

Get Quality Sleep

A good night's sleep is the best way to start your day. As I discussed in Chapter 6, it's very difficult to face a busy day if you start out fatigued and achy due to poor quality or quantity of sleep. Research has shown that sleep rejuvenates and retools the immune, nervous, musculoskeletal and endocrine systems of the body—systems needed to effectively deal with the stresses of everyday life. Review "Prescription for Restful Sleep" in Chapter 6 for practical tips for facilitating good quantity and quality sleep.

Regular Physical Activity

A foremost breakthrough in health research in the past three decades is identifying the role of cortisol, the so-called stress hormone. An important function of this primitive hormone is to keep a person awake, alert and fully cognizant during the day. Cortisol levels are supposed to drop to imperceptible levels at night. However, 21st-century lifestyle, characterized by 24/7 activities and incessant stressors, causes people to produces excessively high levels of cortisol—daytime and nighttime! In fact, some sleep experts partly blame excessive nighttime secretion of cortisol for the steep rise in insomnia.

The best way to lower cortisol and other detrimental stress-related hormones is to engage in daily physical exercise. Regular exercise burns off cortisol, preventing its destructive tendencies. Exercise also mobilizes endorphins—brain-sedating, morphine-like substances that are nature's gift for managing stress!

Anti-Stress Eating

Excess and chronic cortisol secretion induces food cravings—invariably for refined sugars! As you learned in Chapter 2, these macronutrients can trigger an aggressive release of insulin which quickly lowers your circulating blood sugar, causing you to crave more sugar in an attempt to restore your blood sugar to homeostatic levels. Antistress nutrition practices include:

- Chew your food slowly and deliberately to promote healthy digestion, slow transit time of the food through your gut, and prevent overeating.
- Consider taking a probiotic supplement, which can replace friendly gut bacteria and facilitate healthy digestion.
- Eat complex carbohydrates (e.g., whole wheat, whole grains) instead of simple carbohydrates to stabilize your blood sugar.

A drop in blood sugar can trigger the production of stress hormones.

- Consume at least 30 grams of dietary fiber everyday, which can help control weight, blood sugar, and cholesterol.
- Eat at least 5 to 10 servings of vegetables and fruits daily.
- Eat only healthy proteins (e.g., beans and tofu) which are low in calories and can help control hunger pangs.
- Consume only healthy fats (e.g., omega-3 monounsaturated fatty acids) which can enhance mood.
- Stay well hydrated as dehydration can trigger stress hormones. See Chapter 2 for a discussion on how much water you should consume daily.

Form Healthy Social Relationships

People who have strong social support systems are better prepared to deal with stress than their non-connected peers. In Chapter 8, I'll discuss practical approaches to building lasting relationships.

Regarding stress and healthy relationships, intimacy is crucial to optimal wellness. Indeed, a healthy sex life pays huge wellness dividends. Studies after studies have shown that individuals with active sex lives have less overall stress, low rates of insomnia and fewer cases of chronic pain. Oxytocin levels surge just before orgasm, which in turn releases natural pain-killing endorphins. Oxytocin also acts as a natural sedative, facilitating relaxation and deep sleep.

Volunteering to help the less fortunate, without expectations of profit, is a great stress busting technique. Selfless community service to help the less fortunate positively influences one's biochemistry. It also helps to reaffirm that we're one human race and that the happiness of each is connected to the happiness of all!

Volunteer opportunities abound. You can volunteer to feed the homeless or take meals to the shut-in one day a week. Many service organizations are always looking for people to take the elderly or disabled to medical appointments. You can also volunteer to help your own relatives. In the process, you can build and strengthen social ties that can last a lifetime.

Employ Humor

Seeing the funny side of a stressful event or issue is a great way to attenuate its searing effects. The late Norman Cousins, a bestselling author and renowned advocate of the health benefits of humor, left us a huge scientific database supporting the health promoting benefits of happiness through laughter.

In addition to releasing pent-up emotional tension, laughing causes the secretion of endorphins and other stress-busting substances. Laughing sets the stage for a positive perspective that supports healthy thinking and behavior. Additionally, laughing enhances the health of the cardiovascular, gastrointestinal and immune systems.

Practice Relaxation Techniques

An important strategy for dealing with emotional stress is to learn and practice a relaxation technique that fits you. Whichever strategy or strategies you select should be portable, effective, and simple enough to be practiced in between normal daily activities. These modalities include visualization, meditation, progressive muscle relaxation, biofeedback and yoga. Unlike drugs, these modalities are free and their only side effects are improved emotional and physical health—they relax both the body and the mind.

Visualization or Guided Imagery. A long list of behavioral medicine experts like Dr. Herbert Benson of Harvard Medical School, have demonstrated that our thoughts are the foundation of our behavior. The human mind has an amazing capacity to create both positive and negative images that can effectively drive our mood and actions. For example, you may be able to give yourself a headache by thinking of a bad accident scene, or become hungry by thinking about a scrumptious cheesecake.

Similarly, the power of the mind can be harnessed to lower your blood pressure, relax tense muscles and mitigate emotional distress. In visualization, your mind creates your own positive imagery that can also be used to mentally and physically relax. This stress-relieving strategy is easy to learn and master.

First, sit or lie down in a comfortable position and close your eyes. Monitor your body for tenseness and relax as much as possible. Then, visualize a place, scene, or object that is pleasant and soothing. For example, try to remember every detail of a family picnic or camping trip that made you happy. Who was there? What happened? What did you talk about? Savor the sights, sounds, smell, and taste of your experience.

As you become consumed by your experience, your body will relax and your mind clear. You can enhance your experience by whispering positive statements like "I'm feeling very relaxed" or "My mind is crystal clear."

Meditation. During the course of a hectic day, the body becomes stiff and the mind gets agitated. Meditation helps restore calmness and induces relaxation—conditions needed to mitigate stress and its harmful effects. During meditation, heart rate slows, blood pressure drops, the adrenal glands produce less cortisol, and immune function improves.

There are many varieties of meditation practices from which to choose. One of the most common is mindfulness meditation, which helps you to be fully present in all your activities. This makes you more alert and enhances your memory. Mindfulness helps you use all of your senses throughout the day.

To meditate, sit or lie in a relaxed position in a quiet room. Focus on a sound like "ooommm," your own breathing, or nothing at all. Do this for 5 to 15 minutes and you'll feel rejuvenated and ready to handle difficult and unpleasant situations. Like any new skill, mastering meditation will take practice.

Progressive Muscle Relaxation. Designed by the late Dr. Edmund Jacobson of the University of Chicago, this stress-relieving strategy is portable, simple, and easy to learn. You can do it in the privacy of your home or in public. Progressive muscle relaxation involves a two-step maneuver in which you tense and relax different muscle groups. For example, if you want to progressively relax your shoulder muscles, you'd firmly elevate your shoulders, hold for a count of ten, and then relax the muscles.

The best approach to progressive muscle relaxation is to systematically start at your feet and work your way up to the top of your head. After sitting in a comfortable position, breathe slowly and deeply in and out for a few minutes. Take another minute to feel the tenseness in each of your muscles. Finally, start the tense-relax cycle in your feet, legs, thighs, buttocks, abdomen, back, neck, face, and scalp.

Biofeedback. This form of behavioral therapy has roots in the meditation movement of the 1950s and 1960s. Biofeedback allows you to monitor your body's physiological functions (e.g., heart rate, skin temperature, blood pressure and muscle tension) and alter them through operant conditioning.

Using audiovisual aids (e.g., a beeper or flashing light) to see or hear various bodily functions, the individual can use deep relaxation, self-suggestions, and other techniques to voluntarily alter the body function in question. When the feedback light flashes or the beeper beeps too often, the biofeedback trainee must use the learned techniques to alter the audiovisual signals and thus the body functions being monitored.

Biofeedback is usually taught by various healthcare professionals such as social workers, psychologists, psychotherapists and nurses. Check with your primary healthcare provider for a referral to a biofeedback practitioner. Mastering biofeedback requires practice and will take time so don't expect to significantly lower your stress levels after one or two sessions of biofeedback.

Yoga. This form of physical and mental relaxation has its roots in Hinduism, which emphasizes mind-body connection. Originated in Asia over 6,000 years ago, yoga has enjoyed overwhelming popularity in the West in the past two decades. It can help reduce stress by quieting the mind and restoring the mind-body connection.

Tai Chi. More and more, Americans are discovering this ancient, Chinese mind-body modality. At the core of the premise of Tai Chi is the generation of internal energy to balance body, mind and spirit to promote general health and wellness. Indeed, practitioners have reported improvement in muscle tone and cardiovascular, respiratory and digestive disorders.

Although it will take years to master Tai Chi, you can benefit from this Eastern practice from the outset. The best way to learn Tai Chi is to enroll in a class. Other options include many books and DVDs available at bookstores and via Internet retailers.

WHEN ALL ELSE FAILS

This chapter addressed people with everyday stress, not persons with severe forms of anxiety such as phobias, panic attacks, and obsessive-compulsive disorders. These individuals require intense psychotherapy; not the strategies outlined in *Prescription for Wellness*! This is why, throughout this book, I recommend evaluation by a primary care provider to determine the intervention that's best for *you*.

The vast majority of people succeed in managing their stress using the aforementioned strategies. If, despite your best efforts at self-managing your stress, you continue to fall victim to this phenomenon, please seek the help of a qualified healthcare professional specializing in stress management.

Most authorities agree that the most effective treatment for disabling emotional stress is cognitive behavioral therapy (CBT). This form of stress management therapy helps the individual identify *his* sources of stress, restructure priorities, change his or her response to stress, and find practical methods for managing and reducing distress. CBT is especially helpful when the source of stress is chronic pain or other chronic diseases. CBT is taught by a number of healthcare professionals such as social workers, psychologists, psychotherapists and nurses. Check with your primary healthcare provider for a referral to a CBT practitioner.

IN SUMMARY

- Modern lifestyle exposes us to long-term stressors that can be *perceived* as threats to our physical or mental well-being—the genesis of the epidemic of stress, distress and stress-related diseases among Americans.

- Excessive emotional stress incurs a "fight-or-flight" response, characterized by a complex interplay between the nervous system and a series of hormones (called catecholamines) that prepare the body to *physically* deal with the perceived threat.

- Medical researchers have linked chronic psychological distress to the development of a number of physical disorders such as eczema, insomnia, headache, depression, thyroid dysfunction, heart disease, hypertension, ulcers, and overweight and obesity.

- To break your distress cycle you must: identify your stressors; develop healthy ways of thinking; practice mindfulness; establish personal boundaries; get quality sleep; stay physically active; eat healthfully; form healthy social relationships; employ humor; and practice relaxation techniques. When all else fails, see a health practitioner for cognitive behavioral therapy.

Chapter 8

Form Good Social Connections

"When people are asked what pleasures contribute most to happiness, the overwhelming majority rate love, intimacy, and social affiliation above wealth or fame, even above physical health."
—John T. Cacioppo & William Patrick
Co-authors of *Loneliness: Human Nature and the Need for Social Connection*

A little more than a year ago, while bowling at my local bowling center, I witness a poignant event: two young men, who appeared to be friends hanging out for the afternoon, bowling against each other while wearing headphones and enjoying their own recorded music! How sad, I thought—a favorite pastime traditionally punctuated by lively conversation and "high fives" is now relegated to parallel fun! These young men were not being unusual; they demonstrated a sad trend in our society—a growing lack of social connectedness.

Humans are naturally social beings; we are not supposed to be isolated. In our earliest days on earth, we lived in large tribes and communes. We experienced shared safety, pursued common goals, and prescribed to a common purpose. However, as we've become *modern*, we've progressively abandoned our earliest social instincts to pursue isolation—a concept we now call *privacy*. Indeed, many aspects of modern life continually and unavoidably separate us from the social connectivity that's part of our DNA. The nuclear family that defined our original existence has all but disappeared.

A large body of research has shown that social isolation—not having solid social relationships—is an independent risk factor for illness and poor health.[1] Conversely, good social linkages—solid and reciprocal connectivity to others, and positive interactions with social institutions and mores—can help strengthen the immune system and code for overall good health and wellness. You can say that a network of friends and family is similar to good health and life insurance—it's special to have close support in times of trouble!

DANGERS OF SOCIAL DISCONNECTION

Growing up in a close knit family that includes five siblings, 18 year-old Mary fully expected to miss her relatives when she left to attend college, approximately 1500 miles away. From the outset, she struggled to adjust to her new reality. Eventually, she experienced a resurgence of her asthma and eczema that had been quiescent for over 13 years. Mary's roommate considered her a wimp for poorly adjusting to life without the physical presence of her parents and siblings.

Is Mary a weak-minded wimp? Why did she feel so socially disconnected from the people with whom she lived, laughed, fought, and confided for 18 years? What's the connection between separation from her loved ones and Mary's medical problems? Let's examine some of the more significant illnesses related to social disconnections:

Poor Mental Health

A litany of evidence show that socially disconnected persons are at increased risk for anxiety, excessive stress, aggression, memory impairment, age-related cognitive decline and depression. Apparently, social isolation leads to a reduction in production of the brain's neurotransmitters that facilitates healthy brain function.[2]

Heart Disease

Speaking at the 2005 American Heart Association's annual meeting, Dr. Eric Loucks presented a scientific paper showing that men who were socially isolated had elevated levels of inflammatory markers in their blood that signal risks for imminent heart disease. Participants with the lowest levels of social involvement had the highest levels of Interleukin-6, a biomarkers linked to coronary heart disease.[3] How does social disconnection impose a higher risk for heart disease? It seems that people who have poor social connectivity are more likely to engage in unhealthy behaviors such as being sedentary and abusing alcohol.

Immune Dysfunction

In one large study, persons with poor social support systems were found to have elevated levels of cortisol, a hormone recognized as an immune system suppressant. How does this happen? How does social isolation raise cortisol levels?

Chronically elevated cortisol levels are connected to chronic, excessive stress. Additionally, poor sleeping habits can raise cortisol levels. Finally, central obesity (i.e., an elevated waist-to-hip ratio) has been linked to elevated cortisol levels. Excessive emotional stress, insomnia, and overweight and obesity are commonly found in people with a poor network of friends, relatives and other acquaintances.

Early Death

Socially disconnected people die an average 4.5 years earlier than their socially connected peers. Not surprising since social isolation imposes poor mental health, cardiovascular disease and poor immune function, conditions all linked to premature mortality.

STRATEGIES FOR GETTING CONNECTED

Some people are natural at forming friendships and staying connected with friends, relatives and casual acquaintances. They are the life of the party, first to strike up a casual conversation, and great at keeping in touch. As a result, these individuals have no shortage of friends, relatives, and acquaintances with whom to connect. If this is not you, you'll have to learn these social techniques. How can you learn to form and foster enduring social and casual relationships?

Like any other acquired skill, the ability to form and foster social and casual relationships can be learned and mastered. Shy and socially inept individuals whose profession (e.g., politician) or avocation (e.g., community organizer) depends on this ability, learn to master these skills, and so can you. The first thing you should do is to develop a social connectivity plan then work your plan.

Social Connectivity Plan

In your plan, make a list of friends, relatives, co-workers, and other acquaintances (e.g., fellow professionals) with whom you'd like to form enduring relationships and/or just to stay in touch (e.g., a sick aunt who lives alone). Identify those who've been positive and supportive of you in the past.

Next, identify a mechanism for how you'll connect with each person on your list—for example, e-mail every Saturday, call the first Sunday of each month or have brunch the third Sunday of each month. Enter this into your planner as you confirm the other party's availability. Finally, make a solid commitment that you'll stick to your plan, come rain or shine, snow or heat wave!

Connecting with Family and Friends

In this section, I'll talk about creating opportunities to connect with persons on your list and developing a long-term relationship with a "bragging buddy."

Create Opportunities to Connect. In your social connectivity plan you should list strategic opportunities to connect. These can be as simple as going window shopping or as in-depth as organizing a family reunion.

Family team building trips are usually a blast, physically healthy and can help bring family members closer together. Holidays such as Easter, Memorial Day, Labor Day and Thanksgiving offer great opportunities to get together.

Find a "Bragging Buddy." In my wellness practice, I urge all of my patience to cultivate a relationship with a close friend or confidante with whom they can ritualistically get together weekly or monthly. This friendship must be based on openness, uncompromising confidentiality, and mutual admiration. For the most part, bragging buddies should be of the same gender.

During these meetings, both parties can talk about their frustrations, disappointments, wishes, triumphs, and dreams. An important rule for these meetings is that both parties have to be good listeners! My patients tell me that, in addition to being a great stress management technique, having a bragging buddy helps confirm their self-efficacy, solidify their self-esteem, and energizes their spirits.

Connecting to your Community

A common trait among happy people is their connection to their community. During times of stress and family tragedy, socially connected neighbors can provide invaluable support and contribute to one's resiliency. Social clubs, religious activities, and volunteer organizations offer excellent opportunities for community connections.

Join a Social Club. Membership in a social club provides a great opportunity to meet and network with individuals from all walks of life. A large variety of social clubs advocate recreation and activities such as fishing, golfing, politics, and charity work. These clubs attract members from all walks of life and typically facilitate opportunities for a rich social network of friends.

Attend Religious Activities. A 2004 study done at Wake Forest and Emory Universities showed that attending religious services contributed to health as much as quitting smoking or getting more exercise.[4] In addition to promoting mental health, religious activities foster tight relationships based on common interests and beliefs.

Volunteer. As I discussed in Chapter 7, volunteering is a surefire way to mitigate stress and boost your health and wellness. Volunteering helps you to help others and to meet wonderful people. In my wellness practice, I prescribe this as stress management and social connectivity tools and it works—many of my patients are virtually transformed by donating their time to help others!

Volunteer opportunities abound. You can volunteer to feed the homeless or take meals to the shut-in one day a week. Many service organizations are always looking for people to take the elderly or disabled to medical appointments and other activities. You can also volunteer to help your own relatives. In the process, you can build and strengthen social ties that can last a lifetime.

Connecting to your Profession and/or Avocation

As a natural medicine doctor deeply devoted to family, community and profession, I have a busy life! My daily schedule is jam packed with appointments, meetings, social events, and errands. My family time is sacred and untouchable. My community involvement is wide and deep.

Professionally, I keep up with current health trends and new medical discoveries by reading, listening to audio CDs, watching DVDs, and attending medical conferences. However, I rarely get the opportunity to sit down with professional colleagues for intellectual exchanges; they, too, are busy and divide their time between competing priorities.

These challenges notwithstanding, I recently decided to make it a point to set aside one hour each week to meet with a medical colleague to talk shop. I have to tell you that this is one of the best 60 minutes I spend each week! We discuss current medical issues, the politics of medicine, and future trends. These discussions also allow us to voice our opinions on the trends of the American healthcare system and to reaffirm our commitment to the ideals of our profession.

I highly recommend that you commit to spending time with like-minded professionals as often as your schedule will allow. Join your County or State professional society. If you elect to socially connect via your hobby or avocation (i.e., an activity outside your primary occupation), you should be able to find these organizations within close proximity to your home. Examples include bird watching, amateur sports, amateur acting, and genealogy.

The social bonds you can develop through professional or avocational organizations can have profound biopsychosocial benefits. Try it!

IN SUMMARY

- Human beings are naturally meant to be tightly connected socially.
- Numerous scientific studies have clearly demonstrated a link between social relationships and health, wellness and life expectancy.
- The dangers of social isolation include: poor mental health; heart disease and stroke; immune dysfunction; and early death.
- Strategies for getting socially connected include: develop a social connectivity plan; plan to connect with family and friends; develop a plan to connect with your community; and plan to connect with your profession and/or avocation.

Chapter 9

Adopt a Spiritual Belief System

"A bodily disease, which we look upon as whole and entire within itself, may, after all, be but a symptom of some ailment in the spiritual part"
—Nathaniel Hawthorne

The fundamental premise of *Prescription for Wellness* is that humans are necessarily multidimensional: mind, body, and spirit. Scientific medicine has room for the body (i.e., physical health) and the mind (i.e., mental and emotional health) dimensions of our being. However, the concept of the spirit is the antithesis of scientific medicine, which strictly embraces evidence-based concepts only and has no room for faith-based concepts.

Recently, however, medical experts are starting to articulate an interesting clinical observation: patients who live with a profound sense of purpose and meaning (i.e., their spiritual dimension), achieve healthy biochemical milieus. In recent years, also, numerous studies extol the healing powers of prayer and other spiritual practices—some of the oldest healing modalities known to man. Gurus in integrative and holistic medicine such as Dr. Andrew Weil, Dr. Don Colbert, and Dr. Kenneth R. Pelletier write that spirituality is a mandatory ingredient for optimum health and well-being. World-renowned psychologist and modern-day philosopher, Dr. Wayne Dwyer, is noteworthy for saying that humankind are spiritual beings having a human experience rather than the other way around.

Let's now examine what is spirituality, the health benefits of practicing spirituality, and discuss pragmatic tips on how you can adopt a spiritual practice that suits you.

WHAT IS SPIRITUALITY?

One of my medical professors was fond of saying that after studying the human body and gaining full knowledge of its complex and sophisticated design and function, there is no way you can conclude that human creation is an accident! You unavoidably develop the capacity to believe that a supernatural or divine force with unfathomable skill created humankind. The heart, for example, incessantly beats with relatively few pauses, between birth and death! No machine can lay claim to that level of endurance. The marvel of the brain and its ability for cognition makes it a fantastic organ designed with fantastic skill and purpose. So, what does all of this have to do with spirituality?

Spirituality is the deep recognition that there is a universal life force greater than oneself, to borrow a definition from Dr. Kenneth R. Pelletier, Professor at the Stanford University School of Medicine. This life force is beyond the logical comprehension of our five senses. In fact, this life force can only be appreciated via faith—blind belief.

Spirituality is not necessarily religion and not necessarily associated with religion. However, Christianity offers a good example—through faith, Christians believe that Christ, the son of God, was sent to earth to minister to mankind and to give mankind the opportunity for redemption and to achieve everlasting life in heaven. Ritualistically observing an honoring this core aspect of human existence is the centerpiece of Christian belief.

On another level, spirituality recognizes that we have an inner soul that in interconnected to the vast universe via a supernatural force. Our spiritual goal in life is to develop an understanding of human connection to the universe via a divine intelligence and to aim for integration and wholeness. Spiritual growth and development involve the following questions and reflections:

- Who am I?
- What's my purpose for being here on earth?

- With what gifts and skills have I been blessed?
- What's my true level of courage and strength?
- How do I reconcile goodness and suffering?

Spirituality, then, is a growth level of our existence where we find profound meaning in our presence on earth, our life purpose, our relationship to the universe, and the future of our spiritual beingness. Recognizing the power of spirituality has very important application in everyday life: it helps us deal with overwhelming stress; provides inner peace; imparts hope; offers answers about the infinite; helps us find inspiration; and helps us deal with loss and bereavement.

Finally, spirituality is available to everyone regardless of gender, age, national origin or any other sociodemographics—because we are all spiritual beings having a human experience. Indeed, spirituality is an inseparable dimension of human nature.

HEALTH BENEFITS OF SPIRITUALITY

Ancient cultures recognized that spirituality can offer many emotional and physical benefits. Prior to the introduction of modern medicine, physical and mental healing was approached from a spiritual angle. Shamans and medicine men routinely (and relatively successfully) used herbs and spiritual rituals to treat physical and emotional conditions.

Regrettably, our modern culture is only now beginning to recognize the healing benefits of spiritual growth and development. Some authorities predict a spiritual renaissance in the United States. Slowly but surely, we are beginning to realize that spirituality can boost self-esteem, improve overall health, and can contribute to health and longevity.

Boost Self-Esteem

Self-esteem, the mental image we have of ourselves, plays a crucial role in our health and wellness. This self-image influences our thoughts, our relationships, and the choices we make. It has implications for how we function in our workplace, how we deal with others, and how successful we become. In fact, a low self-esteem is a major contributing factor to unhappiness, anxiety, depression, dysfunction, and myriad physical illnesses.

Spiritual practices can boost your self-esteem by providing you with a sense of purpose, meaning and direction. Research shows that adopting a spiritual practice can enhance your self-image leading to heightened creativity, adaptability, flexibility, humility and benevolence.[1]

Good Overall Health

The National Center for Complimentary and Alternative Medicine (NCCAM) is supporting research into the role of spiritual practice and health. Dr. Catherine Stoney, a Program Officer with NCCAM, noted that: "There is already some preliminary evidence for a connection between prayer and related practices and health outcome. For example, we've seen some evidence that religious affiliation and religious practices are associated with health and mortality—in other words, with better health and longer life. Such connections may involve immune function, cardiovascular function and/or physiological changes."

Other research shows that people who describe themselves as spiritual have lower blood pressure, lower rates of depression, and are less likely to engage in self-destructive behaviors such as smoking, using illegal drugs and abusing alcohol.[1]

Longevity

Recent scientific evidence suggests that adoption of a spiritual reference can help an individual achieve low disease burden and even extended life expectancy. In his well-written book, *The Blue Zones*, author Dan Buettner describes that one commonality among centenarians around the globe is their observance of some form of spirituality. For example, the Okinawan centenarians practice worship of their ancestors; the Sardinians and Nicoyans practice Catholicism; and the Seventh-day Adventists of Loma Linda, California practice Trinitarianism.[2]

That religious activities may help lower mortality suggests that this is a viable way to achieve optimum health and longevity. A recent study conducted by Yeshiva University in New York City showed that people who attended weekly religious services, regardless of faith, had a reduced risk of dying by 20 percent compared with people who didn't attend services. The lead author of the study, psychology professor Dr. Eliezer Schnall, suggested that attending services provided a sense of community and support, which translated into less depression.

OPTIONS FOR PRACTICING SPIRITUALITY

Spiritual practices span a wide spectrum of activities from religious to secular rituals. Any activity that quiets the mind, enhances mind-body connections, and forges connectivity between our conscious self and our divine source, can be defined as spiritual. Some people find spirituality through music, art, and gardening. Others engage in prayer, meditation, yoga, Tai-Chi, or volunteer to serve the less fortunate.

Prayer

Practitioners of all of the major religions believe that the act of praying unleashes the power of a divine being—their God. Praying provides comfort in times of distress; reassurance when doubt prevails; and wisdom when solutions evade the human grasp.

Meditation

But religion is only one way to practice spirituality. Meditation quiets the mind allowing it to focus deeply in order to heighten awareness. As I discussed in Chapter 7, there are many varieties of meditation practices from which to choose. One of the most common is mindfulness meditation, which helps you to be fully present in all your activities. This makes you more alert and enhance your memory.

To meditate, sit or lie in a relaxed position in a quiet room. Focus on a sound like "ooommm," your own breathing, or nothing at all. Do this for 5 to 15 minutes and you'll feel rejuvenated and ready to handle difficult and unpleasant situations. Like any new skill, mastering meditation will take practice.

Yoga

As I also discussed in Chapter 7, yoga can create a deep serenity that can provide short-term and long-term health and wellness benefits. This ancient form of physical and mental relaxation has its roots in Hinduism, which emphasizes mind-body connection. Yoga practitioners experience reduced stress via quieting the mind and restoring or strengthening the mind-body connection.

Tai Chi

Tai Chi is rapidly gaining popularity and for good reason: it creates internal energy to balance body, mind and spirit to promote general health and wellness. Indeed, practitioners have reported improvement in muscle tone and cardiovascular, respiratory and digestive disorders. Although it typically takes years to master Tai Chi, you can benefit from this ancient Chinese practice from the outset. The best way to learn Tai Chi is to enroll in a class. Other options include the many books and DVDs available at bookstores and via Internet retailers.

Volunteer

Volunteering, especially to serve the less fortunate, can give you a perspective of seeing yourself in a profound role in the big picture of life.

Perform one random act of kindness every day, as the late-President Ronald Regan had admonished us when he came into office. As I discussed in Chapter 8, there is no greater satisfaction than knowing you helped another human being.

There are plenty of opportunities to volunteer. You can volunteer to feed the homeless or take meals to the shut-in one day a week. Many service organizations are always looking for people to take the elderly or disabled to medical appointments. You can also volunteer to help your own relatives. In the process, you can build and strengthen social ties that can last a lifetime. Moreover, you can advance your spirituality!

Gardening

Gardening is a profoundly spiritual activity! It connects you with nature more than any other activity can. Plants, flowers, the soil and everything associated with gardening can bring you comfort and joy by reminding you that however you think of yourself, you are intimately connect to the natural world.

IN SUMMARY

- Humans are multidimensional: mind, body, spirit. Modern life and scientific medicine (with evidence-based practice at its core), have helped separated us from our spiritual lineage.
- In recent decades, health and philosophy experts are beginning to realize that humans are spiritual beings having a human experience rather than the other way around.
- Spirituality is the deep recognition that there is a universal life force greater than oneself.

- Spiritual practice can boost self-esteem, improve overall health, and can contribute to longevity.
- Some people find spirituality through music, art, and gardening. Others engage in prayer, meditation, yoga, Tai-Chi, or volunteer to help the less fortunate.

Chapter 10

Don't Use Tobacco Products

"One thousand Americans stop smoking every day—by dying!"
—Author Unknown.

The Centers for Disease Control and Prevention estimates that approximately 24 percent of American adults—45 million people—currently use tobacco products. The U.S. Surgeon General characterizes tobacco use as the most *preventable* risk factor for cancer, cardiovascular disease, and overall deaths among Americans. In fact, it is responsible for killing an estimated 500,000 people annually and incurs more than $160 billion in health-related expenses each year.

Tobacco contains over 4,000 harmful chemicals, most of which have been classified as carcinogens. Smokers, chewers, and dippers consume formaldehyde (embalming fluid), acetone (a solvent), cadmium (used in batteries), vinyl chloride (used in plastic), arsenic (a poison) and a litany of other unhealthy substances, with each cigarette, chew or dip. Besides being addictive, nicotine, the active drug in tobacco, is an effective insecticide, used to kill cockroaches and other insects.

WHY DO PEOPLE USE TOBACCO?

Given the foregoing facts, it is quite amazing that anyone would consider using smoked or smokeless tobacco. So, why do people use tobacco? Is it due to a convergence of a complex set social, psychological, and physiological factors?

Any discussion about why people use tobacco should begin with a discussion about why people *start* using tobacco in the first place. Most tobacco users start using tobacco during their pre-teen and teen years. These are turbulent and formative years when youngsters are developing social identities and engaging in behavior patterns that can be characterized as experimental and rebellious. Tobacco is the perfect product to advance a youngster's goal of developing a unique social identity.

The most common reasons people start and continue to use tobacco products include:

Peer Pressure

Surveys of tobacco-using teens reveal a strong need to fit in, which frequently includes using tobacco products. We should fully recognize the omnipresence of peer pressure and the powerful force it is in the lives of our teens! For the typical teen, it's cool to engage in the same behaviors as his or her contemporaries—especially behaviors that are frowned upon by adults. Moreover, teens who march to a different beat are labeled weirdoes, and juvenile pariahs.

Symbolic Behavior

Teenagers who wish to feel "grown-up" often experiment with forbidden substances like alcohol and tobacco as a symbolic gesture of achieving adulthood. Symbolism is a powerful force for a teen and preteen.

Patterned Behavior

Many pre-teens, teens and some young adults start using tobacco out of the desire to emulate their role models. Invariably, these role models include parents, older siblings, close relatives, and relatives. Sometimes, these role models are famous athletes, movie stars, and other public figures.

Stress Mitigation

Adult users smoke, chew, and dip tobacco in order to manage the emotional effects of life's stressors. They reason that tobacco relaxes them and gives them a sense of calm and control. However, physiologically, nicotine is a *stimulant* that increases heart rate and blood pressure and offers anything but relaxation. How does a stimulant offer a calming counter to stress? This is made possible by the power of suggestion; you can derive relaxation from just about any ritualistic behavior honed over time! The stress relieving behaviors of smoking cigarettes also includes taking smoke breaks, inhaling deeply, and socializing with other smokers. Finally, the nicotine relieves stress by attenuating nicotine withdrawal symptoms.

Boredom Management

Tobacco users admit that when there's a lot of downtime, the easiest thing to turn to is tobacco. It is readily available, produces a quick jolt to the system, and allows for a palpable change in pace.

Nicotine Habit

The habit of using tobacco (e.g., the handling and hand-to-mouth rituals of smoking) becomes too deeply ingrained to abolish. Indeed, the repetitive behaviors associated with using tobacco condition the brain, forcing it to make tobacco use an automatic and indispensible action.

An important aspect of the nicotine habit has to do with the triggers that incite the behavior. Tobacco usage is rarely an isolated behavior; it's always connected to another activity or behavior—a trigger. Common triggers include stress, drinking coffee, driving, talking on the telephone and socializing with other tobacco users. Most tobacco cessation experts believe that success in quitting and staying quit is contingent on successful management of your triggers.

Nicotine Addiction

Addiction is a complex physiological phenomenon that involves an addictive substance or behavior, receptor sites in the brain, and neurotransmitters. Nicotine stimulates multiple receptor sites in the brain and creates a number of physiological changes that encourages continued usage.

Once in the blood stream, nicotine travels to the brain where it occupies nicotine receptors and stimulates neurotransmitters (chemical messengers) to communicate its presence to brain cells. The nicotine-brain interaction eventually leads to an uncontrollable dependence on tobacco where stopping produce unpleasant emotional, mental and physical reactions.

THE BODY UNDER THE INFLUENCE OF TOBACCO

Smoked tobacco delivers nicotine (the active drug in tobacco) into the body via the lungs then into the blood stream. Smokeless tobacco goes through the inner lining of the mouth into the bloodstream. Once in the blood, nicotine travels to every cell in the body where it influences most biochemical processes.

Nicotine violates the blood brain barrier—the ultra-selective barrier between the circulating blood and brain tissue that allows few drugs into the brain—and occupies multiple receptor sites. In women, nicotine can be found in breast milk and in mucus from the cervix. During pregnancy, nicotine readily crosses the placenta and permeates the amniotic fluid.

HEALTH CONSEQUENCES OF TOBACCO USE

Using tobacco isn't just a "nasty little habit!" The 1965 US Surgeon General's report linked tobacco use to a number of cancers. Since then, a long list studies have linked tobacco use to diseases of the brain, eye, cardiovascular system, lungs, and bones.

Brain Dysfunction

A study published in the June 2008 issue of *Archives of Internal Medicine* suggests that middle age smokers are at risk for memory and reasoning impairments.[1] Elderly smokers face the prospects of dementia and cognitive decline.

Eye Disease

Nicotine causes a reduction in blood flow to the eyes via narrowing of the tiny capillaries that supply blood to the eyes. In fact, macular degeneration is linked to the use of tobacco products. An article published in September, 2005 in the respected journal *Eye* determined that smokers run two to three times the risk for developing macular degeneration compared with their nonsmoking peers.[2]

High Blood Pressure

Nicotine in tobacco constricts arterioles forcing the heart to work harder in its effort to pump blood throughout the body. The increased workload drives up heart rate and blood pressure. The Multiple Risk Factor Intervention Trial observed that 35 percent of hypertensive men and 33 percent of hypertensive women of all ages were smokers.[3]

Coronary Artery Disease

Nicotine damages the inner lining of blood vessels (a condition referred to as endothelial damage), rendering them susceptible to deposits of cholesterol and other materials. Chronic cholesterol deposition leads to narrowed and hardened arteries, a condition called atherosclerosis. Smoking lowers HDL cholesterol (i.e., the so-called good or heart-protective cholesterol), further compounding a person's risk for coronary heart disease.

People who smoke are also more likely to sustain blood clots in their legs, placing them at greater risk for stroke and heart attack. Indeed, women smokers who take birth control pills have a 20-fold increase in risk for heart attack due to increased tendency for their blood to clot.

Lung Diseases

Smoking damages lung tissue, negatively impacting lung function. Statistics from public health departments show that smokers experience more bronchitis and pneumonia than non-smokers. The vast majority of cases of chronic lung diseases (i.e., emphysema and chronic bronchitis) are caused by cigarette smoke.

Cancers

According to the American Cancer Society, the incidence of cancers of the lungs, mouth, esophagus, and bladder, among others, is much higher in smokers and smokeless tobacco users than their peers who don't use tobacco products.

Osteoporosis

Bone mineral density is a predictor of bone strength and integrity and the risk for fractures. The precise role of tobacco use in causing osteoporosis is currently poorly understood but an analysis of 29 studies showed a significant correlation between tobacco use and osteoporosis—especially among women. One mechanism might be a tobacco-induced reduction in the production of estrogen, a hormone that protects against bone loss.

Other Consequences

Tobacco use reduces blood flow to the blood vessels that feed the skin, robbing the skin of oxygen and other vital nutrients, which leads to premature wrinkles. Tobacco also causes bad breath. Smoking leaves clothes and hair smelling bad. Long-term smokers have yellow fingernails, a less-than-elegant way to enhance one's appearance.

Men who smoke experience much higher rates of erectile dysfunction than men who don't smoke. Speaking of reproductive potential, both men and women smokers suffer from infertility because of their habit: men via under-production of sperms; while women can experience sluggish ovulation and egg function.

Female smokers also undergo natural menopause at a younger age than their nonsmoking counterparts, according to a report from the US Surgeon General's office. Finally, tobacco users can also look forward to a 44 percent higher risk for developing type 2 diabetes compared with nonusers.

BARRIERS TO QUITTING

Most current tobacco users indicate their desire to quit but cite enduring challenges to doing so. The following represents the stumbling blocks to quitting tobacco products:

Nicotine Withdrawal

Like any addictive substances, tobacco cessation produces a long list of unpleasant symptoms including irritability, anxiety, dizziness, depression and fatigue. Some people also experience sleep disturbances, feelings of impatience, and increase in appetite. These are very difficult symptoms to ignore—or tolerate. Even with nicotine cessation aids to temporize the physical symptoms of withdrawal, many individuals succumb to the psychological effects of trying to quit.

Stress

For most users, especially smokers, tobacco is an effective stress management tool. Taking smoke breaks, inhaling deeply, and socializing with other smokers—perfect stress-relieving strategies—are compelling reasons to continue this behavior.

Low Confidence in Succeeding

Most ex-users succeed in quitting after multiple quit attempts. A high probability of failing causes many people to lose confidence and give up after one or two unsuccessful attempts. That's too bad because each attempt imparts additional wisdom and improves one's chances of succeeding, according to tobacco cessation experts.

WHY YOU SHOULD QUIT TOBACCO

Despite heroic efforts to quit, less than three percent of Americans succeed in quitting during a given quit attempt. Considering the psychological and physical symptoms that accompany nicotine withdrawal, why should someone undergo such an ordeal? What does the risk/benefit ratio tell us? The short answer is: kicking the habit is universally beneficial; continue your habit and face incalculable consequences. Let's examine the benefits of quitting:

Improved Health

As I discussed in the opening paragraph, using tobacco is one of the unhealthiest of all negative behaviors. Quitting restores lost health and certainly prevents future diseases and premature death. Most experts agree that ex-users experience progressive restoration in health and well-being. The 1990 Surgeon General's report concluded that former smokers live longer than those who continue to smoke.

Ten years after quitting, the risk of lung cancer among smokers plummets to a risk level similar to people who never smoked! The cardiovascular and pulmonary risks associated with nicotine can add undue burden on the heart and other body systems that regulate blood pressure.

Save Money

Tobacco products are highly taxed and expensive. In some States, the average price for a pack of cigarettes is as high as $10! With skyrocketing healthcare costs and high unemployment, we should all be super-motivated to maintain good health and prevent illnesses.

Positive Role Model

As I discussed earlier, a large number of pre-teens and teens are inspired to start using tobacco by an adult user. Abstaining will send a powerful message to impressionable teens and pre-teens that not using tobacco is the best way to live your life.

Improved Esthetics

The odor created by the use of cigarettes, cigars, and smokeless tobacco products can be repulsive to people who live, work, and associate with the tobacco user. Yellow fingernails are hardly attractive.

THE ART OF QUITTING

Quitting tobacco is a personal experience. Harassment and pressure by spouses and other relatives and friends, is often unhelpful. However, success is deeply embedded in determination, persistence and gritty tenacity. Many have succeeded in kicking the habit and so can you!

Most successful quitters credit outside help such as attendance at tobacco cessation support groups, the use of nicotine replacement patches, and the use of the antidepressant Zyban. Let's examine the merits of the various cessation aids and support systems:

Support Group VS Individual Effort

Many ex-tobacco users credit friends and relatives for the most important support while attempting to quit tobacco. Not surprising since self-esteem, confidence, and strength are derived mostly from our closest relationships. Others who may provide support are co-workers and healthcare professionals. There's no substitute for a supporting cast of well wishers!

Beyond the individual effort, some people enjoy the support of a formal tobacco cessation support group. These groups offer support from others attempting to achieve a similar goal. There are a large variety of cessation support groups available, some are free and some charge a fee.

How do you select from the various tobacco cessation support groups? Which one is more effective? There is no particular standard that govern support groups, but a few generalizations can serve as a guide. Successful support groups typically prescribe to the following characteristics:

- The group leader is trained as a tobacco cessation facilitator. He or she doesn't have to be an ex-tobacco user. It's also not necessary for facilitators to be healthcare providers.
- Group meetings generally last 30 minutes to an hour.
- Programs usually run anywhere from two to six weeks.
- The curriculum usually includes guided discussions on nutrition, physical activity, stress management, behavioral modification, and relapse prevention.

Most tobacco cessation support groups follow a curriculum developed by the American Cancer Society, the American Lung Association, or the American Heart Association. Check with your healthcare provider or county health department for their recommendation for a support group in your area.

Nicotine Replacement Patches

Because nicotine is the addictive substance in tobacco, nicotine replacement patches represent a logical option for quitting for many tobacco users. Placed on the skin, the patch delivers a steady dose of nicotine into the blood stream. The advantage of the steady dose of nicotine is that you avoid the peaks and valleys of smoking.

Sold over the counter, there are a variety of nicotine patches at different strengths on the market today. Most tobacco users who smoke a pack of cigarettes a day should start with the highest strength patch and stay at that level for 2 to 4 week. They then move to the middle strength patch and stay on it for 2 to 4 weeks. Finally, the lowest dose patch is worn for 2 to 4 weeks. Check with your health practitioner for his or her recommendation for wearing the nicotine patch.

Contraindications for using the patch include a history of heart attack, stroke, and uncontrolled high blood pressure. Pregnant and breast feeding women should not wear the nicotine patch. Side effects include rash, tingling and redness in the area where the patch is worn. Some people report vivid dreams if they wear the patch to bed. DO NOT wear the patch if you continue to use tobacco products!

Nicotine Gum

Like the nicotine replacement patch, the nicotine gum provides the body the nicotine it craves. Unlike the nicotine replacement patch, however, the gum represents an active process of replacing nicotine. Therefore, you have to chew the gum in a specific manner in order to extract nicotine.

The gum is fast-acting and short-acting. Available in 2 mg and 4 mg pieces, the nicotine gum offers an answer to the oral fixation that is common in most tobacco users. Contraindications for using the gum include a history of heart attack, stroke, and uncontrolled high blood pressure. Pregnant and breast feeding women should not use nicotine gum. Side effects include a not-so-pleasant taste and hiccups. Acidic drinks and coffee can prevent absorption of nicotine from the gum. DO NOT chew nicotine gum if you continue to use tobacco products!

Nicotine Nasal Spray

A nicotine nasal spray was introduced as a cessation aid in the US in 1996. A major drawback to this product is that many people dislike spraying anything into their nostrils. Side effects of the nicotine nasal spray include nasal and throat irritation, runny nose, and nausea.

Bupropion (Zyban®)

Bupropion or Zyban is an anti-depressant that was found to minimize the symptoms associated with nicotine withdrawal. It helps stabilize the mood swings that are common during attempts to stop using tobacco.

The drug is obtained by prescription and users must be under the care of a healthcare provider. The dose of Bupropion is 150 mg once or twice daily. Contraindications to taking Zyban include a history of seizures, head injury, brain tumor and diabetes. Pregnant or breast feeding women should not take this drug. Anorexia, bulimia and other eating disorders are additional contraindications to taking Zyban.

A major side effect of Zyban is insomnia. This can be avoided by taking the second dose at least six hours before bedtime. Other side effects include dry mouth, rash, and appetite suppression. Bupropion can be used in conjunction with nicotine replacement therapies such as the nicotine gum or patch.

Varenicline (Chantix™)

Chantix or varenicline is a prescription-only medication indicated for use in tobacco cessation. It works by blocking nicotine receptors in the brain, which impede nicotine from attaching to them, thus precluding the euphoria and satisfaction derived from smoking or chewing tobacco. Eventually, the desire to smoke is diminished and ultimately abolished.

The recommended course of Chantix is 12-24 weeks. The most common side effects are nausea, constipation, bloating, and sleep disturbances. Recently, the manufacturer of Chantix reported troubling side effects among users of the drug, namely cases of sleepwalking, anxiety, low blood sugar in diabetics, and suicide. Chantix was not tested in pregnant women and is therefore contraindicated for women who are pregnant, nursing or planning to become pregnant.

Hypnotherapy

In hypnosis, the recipient is offered a subliminal suggestion in order to temporarily suspend his or her usual skepticism. Studies that employ hypnosis for tobacco cessation show mixed results. Some studies show impressive quit rates at 12 months while others report dismal results. In hypnosis, the therapist makes suggestions for not using tobacco and empowers the tobacco user to use this suggestion to beat back the urge to do so. The hypnotherapist also teaches the tobacco user self-hypnotic skills. The first session typically takes one hour and one or two follow-up sessions are required.

Acupuncture

Acupuncture is an ancient Chinese healing art that uses tiny needles on specific areas on the body to treat disease and pain. Like hypnotherapy, the research on acupuncture shows mixed results with regards to its efficacy in helping people quit using tobacco products. In a review of 22 studies, acupuncture was largely ineffective at effecting tobacco cessation.[4] Nonetheless, it might be worth trying if nothing else works.

Other Cessation Options

Using tobacco is typically an obsessive pursuit. Most smokers plan their day around opportunities to light up. Behavioral science experts tell us that the best way to get rid of an unhealthy obsession is to trade it in for a healthy obsession. Indeed, many ex-smokers attribute their success at staying quit to passionately pursuing healthy activities. A common story among ex-users is thrusting themselves into physical activity. Some become competitive marathon runners while others excel at swimming. Remember: ex-tobacco users should always consult a doctor before pursuing any physical activity!

RELAPSE PREVENTION

Like dieting, tobacco cessation is followed by very high rates of relapse. Most individuals relapse within the first six to twelve months of quitting. In fact, because nicotine alters the brain (imposes more nicotine receptors), relapse is a lifelong possibility.

Fortunately, relapses are short-term setbacks for a good number of ex-users. It is important to regard a relapse as a learning experience. If you do relapse, don't beat yourself up—dust yourself off and get back in the saddle! Employ the following strategies to help you to succeed:

Avoid Triggers

The best strategy for preventing relapse is to avoid the sources that trigger *your* desire to light up, dip or chew tobacco. For example, if alcohol is one of your triggers, it is best to abstain from drinking and situations where people are drinking until such time that you no longer have the urge to smoke while drinking. If driving is a trigger, take a different route to work for a few weeks. If coffee is a trigger, switch to tea.

Analyze a Setback

If you do relapse, analyze what caused you to do so. Relapses are invariably due to stress. If it's stress, determine the chronology of events that led up to your backsliding. Start with the thoughts that led you down the relapse path. Remember that every action begins with a thought! Positive thoughts are mandatory for successfully kicking the habit.

Redouble your Efforts

After analyzing why you relapsed, re-commit to quitting and try again. Implement the same behavioral strategies used during your previous quit attempt. Incorporate your analysis into your new cessation effort.

Have a Cessation Aid Handy

I believe that one of the most important strategies for staying quit is to have handy a supply of tobacco cessation product(s) that previously helped you to quit. For example, if you successfully quit using the nicotine patch, carry a supply of patches with you to fend off the desire to smoke, chew, or dip. If you chose the patch as a relapse prevention strategy, the lowest dosed patch is probably all you'd need.

IN SUMMARY

- The approximately 24 percent of American adults (i.e., 45 million people) who currently use tobacco products are at risk for a long list of preventable diseases such as blindness, hypertension, coronary artery disease, lung disease, cancer, and osteoporosis.
- The U.S. Surgeon General characterizes tobacco use as the most preventable risk factor for cancer and cardiovascular disease.
- Barriers to quitting tobacco are significant and include the fear of nicotine withdrawal; excessive stress; and low confidence in succeeding.
- The art of quitting includes: joining a support group; using replacement patches; chewing nicotine gum; using nicotine nasal spray; taking Bupropion; using varenicline; undergoing hypnotherapy; and opting for acupuncture.
- A relapse prevention plan is just as important as a quit plan.

Chapter 11

Limit Your Alcohol Intake

"All excess is ill, but drunkenness is of the worst sort. It spoils health, dismounts the mind, and unmans men. It reveals secrets, is quarrelsome, lascivious, impudent, dangerous and bad."

—William Penn

British religious leader

Alcohol abuse has an epic and tragic history. It has been implicated in the downfall of multiple Egyptian and Chinese dynasties as far back as 1600 BC. Between 460-320 BC, Greek scholars warned of the dangers of excessive alcohol use. In fact, in the 5th century, BC, Plato proposed that no one under the age of 18 should use alcohol; moderate use for persons 19 to 30; and no limits on individuals older than forty. In the 11th century AD, Simeon Seth, a physician in the Byzantine Court, eloquently described the health effects of alcohol and prescribed pomegranate syrup for alcohol-induced cirrhosis of the liver.

Today, heavy alcohol use—generally defined as more than 2 drinks per day for men and 1 drink for women—is a major public health problem that imposes and estimated 100,000 deaths annually. It is responsible for between 20 percent and 40 percent of all hospital admissions. Alcoholics die an average 15 years earlier than their non-alcoholic peers.

Driving while under the influence is a major social problem that leads to nearly 14,000 traffic fatalities annually. Alcohol-related accidents cost taxpayers around $51 billion each year. Alcoholism hurts entire families in ways that rival even the worst tragedies.

WHY DO PEOPLE ABUSE ALCOHOL?

Ethyl alcohol or ethanol, found in liquor, wine and beer, is formed via the fermentation of yeast, sugars and starches. Alcohol is intoxicating, producing euphoria in users. Like any other drug, habitual users become addicted to it and find it most difficult to stop. There are many biopsychosocial reasons people abuse alcohol including, social escape, stress mitigation, peer pressure, symbolic behavior, patterned behavior and alcohol addiction.

Social Escape

One of the most common reasons people start using alcohol is to escape the realities of their lives and forget their troubles. The brain numbing that alcohol induces does suppress memory and gives the illusion that all's right with the world. Obviously, when the stupor wears off, the person returns to confront reality. Invariably, alcohol creates a new, often more treacherous problem to add to the mix of life's troubles.

Another aspect of social escape is drinking to mitigate shyness in social situations. Many alcohol users are anxious when around certain people (e.g., persons of the opposite gender), and they drink alcohol to help them develop the courage and confidence to approach people by whom they are intimidated when sober. Over the long term, however, alcohol induces anxiety, even panic attacks.

Stress Mitigation

According to many chronic alcohol users, alcohol offers stress relief. After a long day, they rationalize, alcohol gives them a buzz, then it helps them relax and escape their stress. As a central nervous system depressant, alcohol doesn't help a person to deal with stress. In reality, the only way alcohol helps a person to deal with stress is its associated ritualism and the opportunity it creates to socialize with other drinkers.

Peer Pressure

Surveys of teenagers who use alcohol show a strong need to fit in, which frequently includes using alcohol products. Some adults also drink to fit in with co-workers, friends and loved ones.

Symbolic Behavior

Teenagers who wish to feel "grown-up" often experiment with forbidden substances like alcohol as a symbolic gesture of achieving the feeling and appearance of adulthood. Many college students engage in binge drinking as part of the rituals of college life.

Patterned Behavior

Many pre-teens and teens and some adults start using alcohol out of the desire to emulate their role models. Invariably, these role models include parents, older siblings and close relatives. Occasionally, these role models are famous athletes, movie stars, and other public figures.

Alcohol Addiction

New users start out consuming a drink or two during a drinking session and eventually escalate their intake in order to achieve the sought-after buzz. Finally, they become addicted and lose control of their alcohol intake—they become alcoholics.

Addiction is a complex physiological phenomenon that involves an addictive substance or behavior, receptor sites in the brain, and neurotransmitters. Alcohol creates a number of physiological changes that encourages repetitive and escalating usage.

Once in the blood stream, alcohol quickly travels to the brain where it stimulates neurotransmitters (chemical messengers) to communicate its presence to brain cells. The alcohol-brain interaction eventually leads to an uncontrollable dependence on alcohol where stopping produces unpleasant emotional, mental and physical reactions.

THE BODY UNDER THE INFLUENCE OF ALCOHOL

After being metabolized by liver enzymes, alcohol is rapidly absorbed into the blood via the stomach and small intestines. Alcohol violates the blood brain barrier—the ultra-selective barrier between the circulating blood and brain tissue that allows few drugs into the brain—and acts as a central nervous system (CNS) depressant.

The intensity of the effects of alcohol on the body depends on the amount of alcohol consumed, age, gender, body mass index, amount and type of food eaten prior to drinking, and the use of concurrent drugs.

Binge drinking, defined as 5 or more drinks on a single occasion for men and 4 or more drinks for women, is more dangerous than daily drinking.

HEALTH CONSEQUENCES OF ALCOHOL ABUSE

Long-term alcohol abuse affects virtually every organ system in the body, most commonly the brain, the skin, circulating blood, and the cardiovascular, gastrointestinal, kidneys, endocrine, bone and reproductive systems. That some alcohol abusers succumb to diseases faster and more severe than others probably is due to differences in genetic predisposition.

Stroke

Excessive alcohol use drives up total and LDL (so-called "bad") cholesterol and triglycerides levels and lowers HDL (so-called "good") cholesterol, setting the stage for disease of the arteries that feed the brain. Eventually, a stroke ensues. Alcohol-induced strokes are also associated with high blood pressure (discussed below).

Brain Disease

New brain imaging techniques have allowed scientists to study the effects of alcohol on brain function and structure. Heavy alcohol use appears to be linked to brain shrinkage that exceeds normal age-related shrinkage. Alcohol-associated shrinkage uniquely involves the areas of the brain responsible for memory and balance.

Chronic, excessive drinking can also lead to alcohol dementia, which impairs learning and other cognitive skills. Excessive alcohol intake impairs neurogenesis, the daily formation of new brain cells that fosters learning and memory.

Alcohol withdrawal can cause Wernicke-Korsakoffs Syndrome, a potentially fatal disorder linked to vitamin B1 deficiency. Alcoholics also can experience delirium tremens, the brain's response to suddenly withdrawing a CNS suppressant. It's important to note that alcoholics should never quit "cold turkey" but should consult their doctor for medicine that can mitigate potentially life-threatening withdrawal symptoms. For information on medications used in conjunction with alcohol cessation, see the section "Drug Treatment of Alcohol Dependence" discussed below.

Dental Diseases

Excessive alcohol intake affects dental health through multiple mechanisms. It is implicated in the development of periodontal disease, recession of gum margins, tooth decay and mouth sores. Compromised oral health can lead to oral cancer.

Alcohol impairs immune function by suppressing the activity of white blood cells, a condition that invites the risk of infection. Alcohol abusers typically have poor nutrition status, with those with the lowest levels of selenium, vitamins A, C, and alpha-carotene intake having the greatest risk for dental diseases.

High Blood Pressure

A large body of research implicates excessive alcohol use in the development of high blood pressure or hypertension. Studies show that men whose daily intake of alcohol beverages exceeds two drinks (i.e., 24 oz beer; 10 oz wine; or 3 oz 80-proof whiskey) and women who exceed one drink are at risk for developing hypertension. Dubbed "the silent killer" high blood pressure is a lethal disease that leads to a number of potentially life-threatening conditions such as stroke and heart attack.

Coronary Artery Disease

While moderate alcohol use protects the cardiovascular system, alcohol abuse poses numerous threats to the heart and blood vessels. The physical stress of long-standing alcoholism causes the heart muscle to enlarge in a condition known as alcohol cardiomyopathy. In this condition, the heart loses its ability to contract, stymieing its pumping capacity. Women are more prone to this condition than are men.

Regular, synchronous contraction of the heart muscle is necessary for its pumping action. An enlarged heart is incapable of this rhythmic requirement. Additionally, heavy alcohol use depletes the electrolytes needed to drive the heart's electrical activity. As a result of these factors, many alcoholics develop heart arrhythmias that can lead to sudden death.

Excessive alcohol use drives up total and LDL (so-called "bad") cholesterol and triglycerides levels and lowers HDL (so-called "good") cholesterol, setting the stage for the development of coronary artery disease.

Liver Disease

The liver is a major organ of the body responsible for a wide range of health functions including detoxification of the blood. Alcohol is a major toxin that presents a huge challenge to the liver; the demand of detoxifying alcohol's toxic elements leaves the liver with less resources to tackle its myriad other functions.

Alcohol-induced liver diseases include alcohol hepatitis, alcohol fatty liver and cirrhosis. Hepatitis, general inflammation of the liver, can negatively impact day-to-day liver function and can lead to long-term scarring. Alcohol causes fat to deposit within liver cells, impairing their normal functions. Liver cirrhosis can lead to blood coagulation dysfunction, retained fluids, jaundice, coma, liver failure and death.

Pancreatitis

The pancreas mainly produces digestive enzymes as well as glucagon and insulin, the latter two which serve to metabolize glucose. A large intake of alcohol over time negatively affects the production and function of pancreatic enzymes and insulin. Pancreatitis can be initially painless for a few years in some individuals before the organ fails.

Endocrine Disease

Under the influence of alcohol, the liver converts testosterone into estrogen in men. Elevated estrogen in men leads to testicular atrophy and enlargement of the breasts. In women who abuse alcohol, the liver converts estrogen into testosterone. Elevated testosterone in women leads to masculinizing features such as facial hair growth and deepening of the voice.

Cancers

When it comes to alcohol and cancer, the studies are mixed: some show a correlation with excessive alcohol use and cancer; others show no correlation. According to the American Cancer Society (ACS), women who consume more than one drink per day are at increased risk for developing breast cancer. The ACS also links esophageal, liver, pancreatic, colorectal, and ovarian cancers to heavy alcohol use.

Osteoporosis

Bone mineral density is a predictor of bone strength and integrity. The precise role of alcohol abuse in causing osteoporosis is currently poorly understood but several epidemiological studies have shown a correlation between alcohol abuse and osteoporosis. One mechanism of the alcohol-bone thinning connection might be alcohol's depletion of hormone, vitamins and minerals needed for bone growth and remodeling. The poor nutrition status of long-standing alcohol abusers is also a contributing factor.

Reproductive Disease

Bothe men and women who abuse alcohol experience higher infertility rates than their sober peers. Male alcoholics have low sperm counts while female alcoholics experience ovulation and egg motility dysfunction. In addition, women who drink alcohol during pregnancy run the risk of giving birth to children with fetal alcohol syndrome—a horrific health condition that sentences its victims to a lifetime of multiple diseases and early death.

SOCIAL CONSEQUENCES OF ALCOHOL ABUSE

Alcohol abuse is a contributing factor in nearly half of all murders, suicides and auto accidents. Drinking and driving is a major public health problem in the United States. It takes many lives and destroys families and communities at all levels of the socioeconomic strata. Alcohol consumption causes bad breath, an esthetically uncomplimentary personal issue!

HOW DO I KNOW IF I HAVE A DRINKING PROBLEM?

The volume of alcohol consumption is one way to tell if you drink too much. Alcohol-related health problems and relationship discord are additional indicators. The best way to objectively quantify your alcohol use is via one of the many alcohol self-administered tests.

Alcohol Self-test

One of the most popular and respected screening tests to determine whether or not a person suffers from alcohol dependence is the CAGE questionnaire. (CAGE is an acronym for four letters in the four questions that comprise the questionnaire). This screening test is considered simple, accurate, portable, and can be self-administered.[1] Scientifically, it is 93 percent specific and 76 percent sensitive in predicting a drinking problem. Take the following CAGE test to see where you stand:

1. *Have you ever felt you should cut down on your drinking?*
    a. Yes
    b. No
2. *Have people annoyed you by criticizing your drinking?*
    a. Yes
    b. No
3. *Have you ever felt bad or guilty about your drinking?*
    a. Yes
    b. No
4. *Have you ever had a drink first thing in the morning to steady your nerves or get rid of a hangover (an eye-opener)?*
    a. Yes
    b. No

Scoring the CAGE Test. One point is allotted to each "yes" answer. A score of two or more points suggests alcohol dependence, for which you should promptly consult your healthcare provider.

Relationship Problems

Problem drinking typically impacts relationships at all levels—family, friends, co-workers, etc. One common demonstration of the negative influence of alcohol is marital discord. Many alcoholics admit to dysfunctional marriages that are marred by violence, economic difficulties, infidelity and divorce.

Health Problems

Alcohol use becomes problematic if it causes the many health conditions I discussed earlier.

WHY YOU SHOULD STOP ABUSING ALCOHOL

Despite heroic efforts to quit alcohol, relatively few heavy drinkers succeed in quitting. Considering the psychological and emotional "benefits" of continued alcohol use versus unpleasant withdrawal symptoms, why should someone undergo the ordeal of quitting? What does the risk/benefit ratio tell us? The short answer is: kicking the habit is far more beneficial than facing the consequences of continuing to use alcohol. Let's examine the health and quality of life benefits of quitting:

Improved Health

As I discussed earlier, using alcohol is one of the unhealthiest of all negative behaviors. Quitting restores lost health and certainly prevents future diseases and premature death. If you are a woman planning to get pregnant, you should know that alcohol pose a grave danger to the developing fetus. Fetal alcohol syndrome is a sad and devastating chapter in the lives of members of the entire family.

Save Money

Alcohol products are highly taxed and expensive. On the low end, if you avoid spending $80 per week, you can save over $4,000 per year—enough for a great vacation for two! With skyrocketing health-care costs, you should be imminently motivated to maintain good health and prevent illnesses. One of the quickest ways to wipe out your hard-earned savings is to succumb to a major illness such as alcohol-induced liver disease. A few visits to the hospital and watch your life savings evaporate!

Positive Role Model

An important self-esteem booster is the knowledge that someone—especially a family member—looks up to you. Conversely, being a source of embarrassment for the family doesn't help one's self-esteem. Quit drinking alcohol; make your family proud!

Most ex-alcohol abusers report that the process of quitting—which requires perseverance and tenacity—is a badge of honor in their lives. Because it's one of the most difficult hurdles to overcome, quitting provides life-long feedback that you can accomplish just about anything.

Improved Esthetics

The physical appearance and subtle behaviors of someone dependent on a product to function in life is an unflattering image. The fetid breath odor created by alcohol can be repulsive to the people who live, work, and associate with the alcohol abuser. The red face and acne rosacea some alcoholics develop are quite unflattering.

THE ART OF QUITTING

Quitting alcohol is a personal experience. Harassment and pressure by spouses and other relatives and friends, is often unhelpful. Like every successful endeavor, quitting alcohol requires personal conviction, a solid plan, plus the total support of family, friends, clergy, doctors, nurses, and other acquaintances.

As I discussed earlier, there are dangers involved in alcohol withdrawal (e.g., delirium tremens and Wernicke-Korsakoffs Syndrome), therefore it's mandatory that you discuss your plan with your primary healthcare provider! If you're at risk, your doctor will prescribe a drug regimen to prevent you from getting into trouble.

Develop a Quitter's Mindset

Heavy alcohol users typically develop certain thinking patterns that allow them to continue their behavior. To quit, you must think differently. Some individuals listen to personal improvement CDs and adopt a verbal mantra or incantation which they repeat to reinforce their conviction that they are on the right track of life.

Begin with the end in mind. Even before you quit, you can visualize your new lifestyle: free from headaches, nausea, chronic muscle pain, and chronic fatigue. You'll be free to enjoy every breath, smell the roses, and live without the burden of an addiction. Savor your new life!

Plan to Quit

Your quit plan should include the what, why, where, and how to quit (see Table 11-1). It should read like a good business plan with as many specifics as possible: dates, times, places, names, methods, etc. Let's map out possible elements that your quit plan should contain.

What. It's important to recognize that you're not quitting a pleasurable endeavor but a burden that has robbed you of life's many pleasures! The journey on which you're about to embark is priority #1! You'll regain your health, prevent future diseases, and enhance your quality of life.

Why. You're determined to stop alcohol because your relationships have suffered, your family is embarrassed by your drunkenness, your career is on hold, your health is threatened, and your quality of life is in shambles. Other important reasons to quit include reducing the risk of injuring yourself and others in an alcohol-related accident.

When. It's important to set a quit date. Most individuals enlist the help of their family, clergy, doctor, or significant other to determine this date. Select a date that's far into the future to allow you to prepare your environment for your new life but not too far out to encourage you to procrastinate.

Where. This element of your plan might contain places to avoid and places to frequent. For example, you might want to avoid the street on which your favorite bar is located. Conversely, you might want to visit a public park for the serenity it offers.

How. This aspect of your plan should discuss the mechanism you'll adopt to facilitate your efforts. For instance, you might want to adopt a comprehensive Wellness Lifestyle Plan: healthy eating; selected supplements; a physical activity program; stress management; etc (see Chapter 1). Additionally, you should plan to monitor your progress. Some people keep a daily diary and some have reported that just the act of tracking their progress was enough to keep them from backsliding.

You might also want to create an environment that's conducive to your new life. Accordingly, you might want to get rid of all drinking paraphernalia (e.g., beer, wine, home bar, etc) that can trigger relapses. Along the same lines, you might want to stay away from drinking buddies until such time that you feel strong enough to visit with them without triggering the desire to drink.

Studies that evaluate hypnosis for alcohol cessation show mixed results. Some studies show impressive quit rates at 12 months while others record dismal results. In hypnosis, the therapist makes suggestions for not using alcohol and empowers the drinker to use this suggestion. The hypnotherapist also teaches the user self-hypnotic skills. The first session typically takes one hour and one or two follow up sessions are required. Ask your doctor if hypnotherapy is something you should consider.

Acupuncture is another option for some. It's an ancient Chinese healing art that uses thin needles on specific areas on the body to treat disease and pain. Like hypnotherapy, the research on acupuncture shows mixed results with regards to its efficacy in helping people quit using alcohol. Discuss this option with your doctor, as well.

Table 11-1
Alcohol Quit Plan

NAME:
I will quit drinking alcohol on:
My reasons for quitting are:
I have the support of the following persons:
When offered a drink, I will say:
I will adopt a comprehensive wellness lifestyle as follows:
I will join the following support group:
I will track my progress daily by:
I will reward myself by:

Support Group VS Individual Effort

Many alcoholics say that the most important support they received while attempting to quit came from friends and relatives. Not surprising since self-esteem, confidence, and strength are derived mostly from our closest relationships. Co-workers, clergy and healthcare professionals can also provide invaluable support.

Beyond the individual effort, some people do prefer a formal support group. The advantage of such a group is the support you derive from others attempting to achieve the same goal. There are many types of alcohol cessation support groups available, the most popular being Alcoholics Anonymous (AA). There's a good chance that there's an AA support group in your hometown. Ask your doctor, psychologist or social worker to help you locate a support group.

Not all support groups are created equal. Successful support groups typically prescribe to the following characteristics:

- The group leader is trained as an alcohol cessation facilitator. He or she doesn't have to be an ex-alcohol user. It is also not necessary for facilitators to be healthcare providers.
- Group meetings generally last 30 minutes to an hour.
- Programs usually run anywhere from two to six weeks.
- The curriculum usually includes guided discussions on nutrition, physical activity, stress management, behavioral modification, and relapse prevention.

There are also many on-line support forums available. A popular one is The Sober Recovery Community located at: www.soberrecovery.com/forums.

Find a New Hobby

For the heavy drinker, using alcohol is a fun and emotionally rewarding obsession. When you quit, these positive emotions still need to be fed. An important way to stay quit is to find a new but healthy obsession—a hobby. Think of a hobby or avocation that you've always wanted to pursue but never had the time to pursue.

Reward Yourself

An important strategy for recognizing your major accomplishments is to reward yourself. As I said earlier, if you avoid spending $80 per week, you can save over $4,000 per year—enough for a great vacation for two to an exotic place!

Drug Treatment of Alcohol Dependence

Drug treatment of alcohol dependence is complicated and beyond the scope of this book. I would mention that the most common agent used currently to support alcohol cessation is disulfiram. A recent study credits baclofen, a muscle relaxant and antispastic agent, with reducing the craving for alcohol in a cohort of patients with alcohol-induced liver disease. Check with your doctor for his or her approach to drugs to facilitate alcohol cessation.

RELAPSE PREVENTION

Like dieting and smoking, alcohol cessation is followed by very high rates of relapse. Most individuals relapse within the first six to twelve months of cessation. It is important to regard a relapse as a learning experience.

Analyze What Happened

If you do relapse, analyze what caused you to do so. Relapses are invariably due to stress. If it's stress, determine the chronology of events that led up to your backsliding. Start with your thoughts that led you down the relapse path. Remember that every action is preceded by a thought!

Redouble your Efforts

After analyzing why you relapsed, re-commit to quitting and try again. Implement the same behavioral strategies used during your previous quit attempt.

IN SUMMARY

- There are many reasons to stop abusing alcohol, not the least of which is to regain and/or improve your health and quality of life.
- Quitting long-term alcohol abuse must be done under medical supervision due to the potentially fatal sides effects of alcohol withdrawal.
- A comprehensive quit plan is mandatory if you want to successfully stay sober.
- Most ex-alcoholics credit support from friends, family, clergy and attendance at a support group for their success.

Chapter 12

Detoxify for Optimal Health

"Most people are toxic to some degree—and I don't mean their personalities, but their physical bodies. Everyone has toxins stored in his or her body."
—Dr. Don Colbert
Best-selling author of *The Seven Pillars of Health*

In the past 100 years or so, industrialization, technological advancements, and environmental ambivalence have resulted in widespread pollution of our air, water, food and soil. Insecticides, pesticides, herbicides, hormones, radiation, and other toxins are now ubiquitous and considered a normal and enduring part of modern life. Canned foods, aluminum foil, aluminum pans, plastic packaging, pharmaceutical drugs, and mercury amalgam fillings add to our toxic burden. Finally, toxic substances accumulate in the body in response to emotional stress, chronic diseases (e.g., fibromyalgia and rheumatoid arthritis), and as a result of normal metabolism.

The US Environmental Protection Agency estimates that seven billion pounds of toxic waste containing over 80,000 different toxic substances pollute our atmosphere! These environmental toxins inevitably enter our bodies via food, water, and air. Like rust accumulating in pipes, high levels of external toxins accumulate in organs and soft tissues, overwhelming our body's natural detoxification mechanisms. In their New York Times bestselling book, *Ultraprevention*, Drs. Mark Hyman and Mark Liponis write that 100 percent of beef is contaminated with DDT as well as 83 percent of processed cheese, hot dogs, bologna, turkey and ice cream.[1]

Environmental scientists have catalogued the health toll these toxins impose on us. For example, heavy metal toxicity has been linked to Alzheimer's and Parkinson's diseases. The relatively high prevalence of Parkinson's disease among farmers is felt to be related to their high exposure to pesticides. High levels of mercury exposure can affect thyroid function. Researchers now link antibiotic-resistant bacteria in humans to the widespread use of antibiotics in livestock (in addition to the widespread use of antibiotics in humans to treat infections).

Currently, there is near consensus among natural health practitioners that we should periodically detoxify from the outside to augment our internal detoxification and elimination systems.

WHAT IS DETOXIFICATION?

Detoxification, or detox for short, is the process of eliminating toxic substances from the body. The human body is constantly engaged in the removal of retained waste products to maintain health—indeed, to maintain life! This is done via:

- The skin—contains sweat glands that help remove lactate, urea, heavy metals and other materials from the body
- The lungs—removes carbon dioxide and other volatile gases from the blood
- The liver—the workhorse of our detoxification system, detoxifies drugs, filters bacteria from the blood, etc
- The gastrointestinal tract—stool formation and elimination
- The kidneys—filters the blood and eliminates toxic substances in the urine
- The lymphatic system—plays a vital role in immunity, plus it returns fluid that ends up between the body's cells back into the blood stream

Practiced for centuries dating back to ancient Egypt and Greece, detoxification rids the body of retained toxins that elude the body's own cleansing systems. Detoxification aims to cleanse the lungs, liver, kidneys, and blood of excess pollutants. Detoxification experts, such as Dr. Elson Haas of the Preventive Medical Center of Marin in San Rafael, California, recommend that we periodically employ external detoxification strategies for optimal health.

People who undergo periodic detoxification report improved general health, sleep patterns, cognitive acuity, physical appearance, energy level, and digestion. Additionally, detoxification has been credited with fostering successful aging and longevity.

SIGNS AND SYMPTOMS OF SYSTEMIC TOXICITY

The resiliency of the human body often pacifies the full effects of retained toxic metabolites. In spite of its toxic burden, the body manages to perform most biochemical functions—albeit sub-optimally! When the body's natural detoxification mechanisms are overwhelmed, we develop a long list of systemic ailments, such as:

- Skin rashes, boils, and pimples
- Brittle nails and hair
- Unexplained headaches
- Failing memory
- Fatigue and low energy
- Diffuse aches and pains
- Allergies and sinus congestion
- Frequent colds
- Bad breath

- Weight gain
- Food intolerance
- Poor digestion
- Increased flatulence
- Constipation
- Unexplained back pain

WHAT IS YOUR TOXIC BURDEN?

The first step in determining your level of toxicity—your toxic burden—is to visit a natural medicine practitioner versed in detoxification and cleansing. The practitioner will take a thorough history and perform a complete physical examination. He or she will then order select laboratory tests to determine your overall health and toxicity profile. At the follow up visit, you'll review your laboratory results and your doctor will prescribe a customized detoxification program.

Let's now take a look at various aspects of the detoxification evaluation and treatment:

Hair Mineral Analysis

Heavy metal toxicity is more common than is typically portrayed. People who work in certain industries are prone to mineral retention. These occupations include metal work, welding, mining, and battery production. The same goes for people who are exposed to ambient environmental pollutants, such as those living and working in large cities.

Retained toxic minerals settle in our hair and reflect the mineral content of the body's tissues and organs. Excess minerals found in hair include:

- Aluminum
- Antimony
- Arsenic
- Barium
- Bismuth
- Cadmium
- Copper
- Gadolinium
- Gallium
- Germanium
- Lead
- Lithium
- Mercury
- Nickel
- Palladium
- Rhodium
- Tellurium
- Thallium
- Thorium
- Tin
- Tungsten
- Uranium

The hair analysis involves collecting a sample of scalp or pubic hair and sending it in to an approved laboratory for evaluation. Results are generally available in 2 to 4 weeks. See Appendix I for contact information.

DETOXIFICATION PROGRAM

There are numerous forms of external detoxification, all following three basic tenets: cleansing, rebuilding and maintenance. However, each program differs in its intent and action. Some detoxification program aims to cleanse the lungs, liver, or bowel. Others are meant to cleanse the skin and kidneys. I'll discuss a comprehensive regimen that combines all detox programs.

Detoxification specialists recommend that you proceed slowly when detoxifying or run the risk of developing a Herxheimer Reaction, a condition where retained toxins are released faster than the body can jettison them. Signs of a Herxheimer Reaction include headache, nausea, vomiting, and fatigue. See Appendix I for suggestions for individual detox programs.

Healthy Lifestyle

The best detoxifying strategy is prevention of toxic accumulations via avoidance and adhering to a healthy lifestyle. This includes: eating fresh, organic foods; managing your stress; getting quality sleep; drinking healthy, alkaline water; and living in a place where the air, water and soil are not polluted. A healthy lifestyle also includes getting enough sunshine to make vitamin D, currently accorded super-vitamin status for its indispensible role in health promotion and disease prevention. Please refer to previous and subsequent chapters that address each of these elements of healthy aging.

Fasting

Fasting stops the importation of new toxins and allows the body to focus on reducing its current toxic burden. Fasting can last from one to several days.

Juice Fasting

Juicing is more than drinking juice! It involves strategically drinking a variety of organic juices to augment the litany of biochemical processes in the body. Juicing supplies the body with enzymes, vitamins, minerals, and phytonutrients to help it cleanse itself of toxins and re-assert its natural healing abilities. Organic vegetable juice is better for you because it contains more minerals and less sugar than fruit juice.

Most authorities recommend to start low and to go slow. Initially, you should drink one 10-ounce glass of green vegetable juice daily. Green juice has chlorophyll, which can help chelate heavy metals.

Hydration

An important detoxification strategy is to maintain good hydration. As I discussed in Chapter 2, an estimated 65 to 75 percent of the adult human body is composed of water; children's bodies comprise between 85 and 90 percent water, depending on age. Water serves many crucial functions including: regulating body temperature; lubricating joints; facilitating most biochemical processes (e.g., hormone and neurotransmitter production); and serving as a media for transporting nutrients throughout the body. Select one of three ways to ensure adequate hydration: (1) drink eight 12-ounce glasses of healthy fluids (mostly, water), daily; (2) drink enough to ensure that your urine is clear; or, (3) drink enough healthy fluids to make you urinate every 3 to 4 hours.

Saunas & Steam Bath

Sweating via steam baths and saunas are great ways to push toxins out of the body. Please be safe when using saunas; adhere to the posted time limits and restrictions based on health history.

Cleansing Bath

Add ½ cup baking soda, Epsom salt or sea salt to your bath water. Soak for 15 to 20 minutes. The water will turn murky if you eliminate heavy metals such as aluminum and mercury.

Heavy Metal Chelation

There are a number of methods to chelate heavy metals. The most effective way is through the use of the synthetic amino acid, EDTA, which binds well with mercury, lead, cadmium and other heavy metals. Discuss this approach with your natural medicine doctor.

Herbal Detox

Herbal cleansers offer a great way to stimulate the lungs, liver and kidneys. Herbs are powerful medicine so herbal detoxification should be done under the supervision of an experienced herbalist or naturopath.

Slippery elm, comfrey, and senega are good herbs to detoxify the lungs. Dandelion, red beet, parsley, chamomile, black Cohosh, and goldenrod work well to cleanse the liver. Parsley, dandelion, uva ursi, goldenseal and ginger are great kidney detoxifiers.

IN SUMMARY

- Insecticides, pesticides, herbicides, and other toxins are ubiquitous and considered a normal and enduring part of modern life—a legacy of industrialization, technological advancements, and environmental ambivalence.
- These toxins make it into the body via the food we eat, the water we drink and the air we breathe.
- The body's natural detoxification systems—the skin, lungs, liver, gastrointestinal tract, immune system, and the kidneys—can handle a reasonable amount of toxic load but is overwhelmed by today's phenomenally high levels of toxic burden.
- Periodic external detoxification and cleansing is recommended as a way to augment the body's natural detoxification mechanisms.
- Systemic ailments that indicate toxicity include: skin rashes; brittle nails; headaches; poor memory; and fatigue. Other symptoms include: diffuse aches and pains; allergies; bad breath; poor digestion; increased flatulence; constipation; and unexplained back pain.
- A comprehensive detoxification program begins with avoidance of toxins and adhering to a healthy lifestyle. Other strategies include: hydration, fasting, juicing, saunas and cleansing baths.

Chapter 13

Partner With Your Healthcare Providers

"Although in the past decade many medical schools have worked diligently to teach doctors-in-training the importance of listening to patients, it is nonetheless important for patients to acquire their own "bedside manner" to equalize the power imbalance inherent in the doctor-patient relationship"

—Dr. Zeev Neuwirth

Patient-physician communication expert

The current state of the practitioner-patients relationship is abysmal! In the typical healthcare encounter, both the patient and the provider have the same goals in mind—to restore and/or maintain health. Similar goals notwithstanding, the process invariably seems to take on an "us against them" tone! Why is this the case and how did we get into this mess? What can be done to better align the behavior of the patient and the practitioner? How to achieve a win-win healthcare encounter?

To be sure, there's no shortage of opinions as why the practitioner-patients relationship is broken. Some experts blame healthcare providers; others blame patients; yet, others blame insurance companies and the managed-care approach to healthcare delivery.

In this chapter, I'll offer my analysis—a synthesis of many opinions—of what went wrong. I'll also discuss the qualities and expectations that both patient and practitioner should bring to the table to lay the groundwork for a solid partnership. Finally, I'll lay out a survival guide that can help you—the patient—to maximize your healthcare experience, despite the challenges of today's healthcare system.

BARRIERS TO A GOOD PRACTITIONER-PATIENT PARTNERSHIP

The best way to receive excellent care is to develop solid relationships with your healthcare providers. Like any other successful relationship, a good patient-healthcare provider relationship should be founded on openness, mutual trust and good communication. Are healthcare workers open-minded, trustworthy, and good communicators? How about patients—are they holding up their end of the bargain?

In national surveys, healthcare practitioners continue to receive some of the highest ratings on respect and trust. Physicians, arguably leaders of the healthcare team, are held in high esteem and in many cases revered. Despite high marks, some patients label doctors as discourteous, hurried and poor listeners.

On the other hand, healthcare professionals—the default judges of patients—often rate patients as demanding and unreasonable! In one survey, doctors rated 15 percent of their patients as "difficult."[1] Why is disharmony so high between patients and healthcare providers?

Most expert blame the following factors for driving a wedge between patients and their caregivers:

- Scientific medicine that gives doctors and others the aura of being human mechanics, trained to fix broken bodies.
- Managed care, which emphasizes cost-cutting measures such as shorter and shorter office visits and higher provider productivity.
- Managed care, which has reduced healthcare to a commodity and patients to being customers—the quintessential impersonal business arrangement.
- Insurance companies that dictate the practice of medicine and are seemingly arbitrary and capricious in their reimbursement decisions.

- The litigious society that we have become, which pits health workers (potential defendants) against patients (potential litigants).

Despite these realities and challenges, the practitioner-patient interaction can prove to be rewarding for both parties. For this to happen, however, both parties must remain committed to their roles: doctors and other health providers must display the characteristics that patients' desire and deserve; patients must embrace their responsibilities and have realistic expectations of the healthcare encounter.

QUALITIES OF A GOOD HEALTHCARE PRACTITIONER

As leaders in the healthcare encounter, physicians, physician assistants/associates, nurses, pharmacists, chiropractors, physical therapists, dietitians and other providers should take the lead in setting the tone for a patient-centered partnership. What are the universally expected characteristics (i.e., attitudes, demeanor and aptitude) of a good healthcare provider?

The following attributes are generally expected of professionals who deliver healthcare:

Professional Qualification

The public expects healthcare workers to be qualified to deliver the care they provide. For example, podiatrists are expected to have complete knowledge of the foot and ankle and current standards of foot and ankle care. Beyond entry level knowledge, health professionals are expected to maintain competence by staying abreast of the numerous scientific changes that occur in his/her profession and specialty. Continuing education is obtained by attending medical conferences and seminars, listening to pre-recorded audio CDs and tapes, and reading journal articles.

Professionalism

Professionalism has to do with embracing the highest ethical, moral and legal standards of your profession. Included are protecting patients' rights, privacy and modesty. Patients have the right to quality care—the safest, most effective measures to maintain and/or restore health.

Patients' privacy is at the core of the healthcare interaction. It permits the patient to honestly and completely share his/her information with the care provider. Patients invariably feel vulnerable during a health encounter. Maintaining their modesty helps preserve some sense of autonomy and self-esteem.

Good Bedside Manners

Society has always expected good "bedside manners" from doctors, nurses and others bestowed with the privilege of delivering health services to the public. Bedside manners refer to the sum total of all interactive acumen: good communication skills; the display of empathy and sympathy; and tolerance of patients' values. Arrogance, overconfidence, and aloofness exemplify poor bedside manners.

In a study published in a leading medical journal, 72 percent of doctors interrupted their patients' opening statements after an average of 23 seconds.[2] Despite being busy and the linear nature of taking a health history, providers should be good listeners as well as display the ability to explain health concepts clearly and concisely to patients and their loved ones. A good healthcare provider also encourages patients and loved ones to ask questions. Patients also expect their providers to return phone calls in a timely manner.

Health workers often underestimate the amount of empathy and sympathy they display. Empathy is the ability to deeply understand the experience of another person and being able to communicate this understanding: "I feel your pain!" Sympathy is showing deep compassion, exemplified by a willingness to say: "I'm sorry you are suffering!"

Tolerance is accepting someone for who they are and what they represent. Patients come in all colors, races, creeds, and backgrounds; they have disparate values; and their expectations vary. Doctors and other health workers should be tolerant of each patient and work assiduously to restore or maintain the health of all patients despite their demographics or beliefs. A perfect example of this is military combat medics who treat enemy combatants with the same diligence as friendly forces.

Sense of Responsibility

Providers should have a strong sense of responsibility to his/her patients and the profession he/she practices. This motivates the provider to rise to "the call of duty" and to go above-and-beyond in advocating for his/her patients. A strong sense of responsibility is what keeps the health professional going when he/she is physically mentally and emotionally spent. It motivates him/her to sublimate personal gains for the good of his/her patients.

Integrity

Integrity is doing the right thing when no one is looking. Patients expect health professionals to be ethically, morally and legally forthright even when no one is monitoring their actions. This character quality motivates the provider to do the best possible thing for patients under his/her care. An important part of this is providing informed consent—unequivocally and completely explaining procedures and treatments before performing or dispensing them.

PATIENTS' RESPONSIBILITIES

Like any mutually satisfying relationship, patients—the recipients of health services—also have important responsibilities. In spite of the fact that patients don't attend formal education programs (i.e., akin to medical or nursing school) they can easily learn their crucial role in the healthcare encounter. To ensure practitioner-patient collaboration, patients should display the following attributes:

Provide a Concise, But Complete Health History

Every health encounter begins with the doctor's question: *What brings you in today?* With the time constraints imposed by managed care, you can get the best bang for your buck, so to speak, by learning to get to the point. Doctors are trained to solicit a health history along the following lines:

- The chief complaint (What's the basic reason for the health visit).
- Duration of the problem (i.e., how long has a given problem been occurring) and any history of this and related problems.
- The location of the problem (e.g., where does it hurt, and does the pain radiate to another location).
- Description of symptoms and associated symptoms the problem produces (e.g., a sharp pain that induces nausea).
- Factors that make the symptoms better or worse (e.g., pain medication makes it better; noise makes it worse).
- A family history of this or similar problems (e.g., mother with similarly debilitating headaches).
- The names and doses of all drugs and supplements (i.e., vitamins, minerals, and herbs) the patient is taking.

Follow-up visits are less structured and typically deal with improvements, new symptoms, side effects, etc.

Exercise Patience

Healthcare is a high-volume, fast-paced service. With so many people getting sick and injured, there is no such thing as an empty waiting room. Getting angry will not help you and might cause you to appear antagonistic, which can influence the quality of the care you receive and your satisfaction with the healthcare outcome.

Have Realistic Expectations

For patients, one of the most frustrating aspects of healthcare is not being seen at their appointed time. This is perfectly understandable—you've taken sick leave, caught in an unpleasant environment, and your symptoms cause physical and emotional discomfort.

The duration of a healthcare visit is very unpredictable. The asthmatic patient who was appointed prior to your appointed time, may take a few extra nebulizer treatments to stabilize before being discharged, causing your appointment time to be pushed back. Some days are full of these unexpected twists and turns; others go smoothly.

Finally, have the right expectations of healthcare providers and health facilities. Practitioners are very busy people and clinics and hospitals are crowded, noisy places, abuzz with activity. Expect that health workers will appear somewhat hurried (but they should never create an atmosphere of impatience). Don't expect serenity while at a hospital!

Learn About Your Disease or Injury

I'm continually amazed at patients' lack of knowledge of conditions from which they've suffered for many years! Knowledge is powerful medicine! It also facilitates and strengthens the practitioner-patient bond and makes you a pro-active partner in your care. Even a cursory understanding of your condition will make it easier to understand your provider's discussion of the topic. It will also help you to ask the right questions.

Knowledge of your condition will also help you to better select from the various treatment options your provider might recommend. Further, knowledge of your condition can help motivate you to be compliant with recommended management.

Be Willing to Make Concessions

In any successful partnership, both parties must be willing to make concessions. Patients and providers are going to have to be flexible and be prepared to compromise. For example, if you have multiple complaints during a visit when the doctor is 30 minutes behind schedule, negotiate with the doctor to take care of the two most serious problems and return another day to discuss the others. This win-win arrangement accommodates the doctor's challenges and gets you the best care, given the circumstances. The next visit will most likely start out with mutual respect and admiration.

OPTIMIZE YOUR HEALTHCARE VISIT

During a lifetime, the typical adult will encounter a large number of health professionals such as physicians, physician/associates assistants, nurse practitioners, chiropractors, nurses, pharmacists, physical therapists, and occupational therapists. Others who provide health-related services include acupuncturists, dietitians, massage therapists, social workers and genetic counselors. Despite the wide spectrum of care they provide, these professionals have one goal in common: to restore and/or maintain patients' health.

Yet, patients' commonly leave providers' offices with unanswered questions and are poorly motivated to do their part to restore and/or maintain their health. As a patient, what can you do to maximize your healthcare visit, to leave the provider's office motivated and committed to hold up your end of the bargain?

Here are some important strategies you can employ to optimize your satisfaction with the healthcare encounter:

Prepare For the Office Visit

Like anything else in life, preparation helps ensure success. The first step in preparation is arming yourself with as much knowledge of your disease as possible. Next, make a list of questions you'd like answered. List any concerns you'd like to discuss with your doctor, nurse, or pharmacist. Don't forget to bring your insurance card and other paperwork, if applicable.

Submit Your Health History & Questions Before Your Visit

A common complaint of patients is leaving their doctors' offices more confused than when they arrived! Invariably, their confusion is due to the short duration of the visit; difficulty understanding medical jargon; and reluctance to question the doctor. Submitting your health history and your questions to your doctor (via the nurse, if this is more appropriate) before the day of your visit can help eliminate confusion and save time. Don't worry if your questions sound silly to you; if they're important enough to be asked, they're important enough for your doctor to answer them.

The health history will help the practitioner zero in on the most important aspects of your health. With your questions in front of him or her, the doctor can better target his or her discussion. If your questions are not completely answered, speak up—ask the doctor to explain his or her answers in simpler or different terms.

Be Prepared to Be a Co-partner

Many health experts believe that both the care provider and the patient should share responsibility for weighing risks and benefits when deciding on diagnostic testing and interventions. Patients generally need to be educated by the provider before they can be effective co-partners—they need good informed consent.

It might be helpful to read up on the health conditions that concern you prior to your visit. This will give you a basic understanding before the doctor's explanation. It will make you a first-class co-partner!

Take Written Notes During the Visit

Typically, multiple recommendations are made during a doctor's visit. Additionally, the recommendations are technical in nature. Writing down each recommendation and additional notes will help you to better assimilate the information flow. Your written notes can also serve as a roadmap as you implement each recommendation. Alternatively, you can ask your provider for printed materials on the subjects discussed. Knowing that you'll be given written instructions can improve your learning as you'll not have to focus on writing new information during the healthcare visit.

Schedule a Follow-up Visit

If your doctor identifies a problem and makes recommendations for fixing the problem, it's best to make a return visit to determine if your efforts succeeded in fixing the problem. Oftentimes, a follow-up laboratory or radiographic study is needed to make this determination.

IN SUMMARY

- Despite similar goals—to restore and/or maintain health—patients and health practitioners have staked out positions in a senseless, "us against them" standoff.
- Some experts blame healthcare providers for a broken practitioner-patient relationship; others blame patients; yet, others blame insurance companies and the managed-care approach to healthcare delivery.
- There's no denying that the managed-care system, scientific

medicine, and the litigious nature of our society share blame for influencing the breakdown in the provider-patient partnership.

- To restore the provider-patient relationship, practitioners should possess the following attributes: be professionally qualified; display professionalism; show good bedside manners; have a sense of responsibility; and possess high integrity.
- For their part, patients should: learn to provide a concise, yet complete health history; exercise patience; have realistic expectations; learn all they can about their disease and injury; and be willing to make concessions.
- Strategies for optimizing your satisfaction with the healthcare encounter include: prepare for the visit; submit your health history and questions before your visit; be prepared to be a co-partner; take written notes; and schedule a follow-up visit.

Chapter 14

Periodic Health Assessments for Women

"Preventive services for the early detection of disease have also been associated with dramatic reductions in morbidity and mortality."

—Statement in a report from Centers for Disease Control and Prevention

In the 1920s, the American Medical Association (AMA) recommended annual health screenings for healthy adults. Prior to that, people went to the doctor only when they were sick or injured. The impetus for the AMA's recommendation was to identify risk factors and diseases in their early, more treatable stages. However, while the AMA's intentions were noble, the extent of the annual check-up was never fully defined. There was never consensus on its value.

The practice of the annual health examination fell into disrepute as the cost of healthcare began to climb in the 1970s. Clinicians began questioning the return on investment as the majority of these evaluations turned up relatively little pathology (at that time). In Japan, where health promotion and disease prevention are the primary goals of the healthcare system, a relatively normal evaluation serves to reinforce good health habits, and that the *healthcare* system is doing its job to keep citizens healthy. In the US, a normal health evaluation is considered by "disease-fighters"—members of our current *sickcare* system—to be a waste of money.

In the 1970s the Canadian Task Force on the Periodic Health Examination (CTFPHE) was formed to evaluate the wisdom of the periodic health examination and to make recommendations for future health check-ups. In 1984, the United States Preventive Services Task Force (USPSTF) was formed with mandates similar to its Canadian counterpart. Today, both task forces serve vital roles in helping to define the periodic health examination—the CTFPHE for a true *healthcare* system and the USPSTF for a true *sickcare* system.

In addition to the CTFPHE and the USPSTF, public health agencies, patient advocacy groups and medical specialty organizations such as the American Academy of Family Physicians and the American Academy of Obstetrics and Gynecology promulgate position papers that spell out their recommendations for periodic health screenings for apparently healthy people. A 2007 study found widespread value of the periodic health evaluation.[1]

In this Chapter, I'll synthesize the current recommendations of various advocates for screening apparently healthy adult women. Because each patient is unique with her own needs, I strongly recommend that you consult your doctor and other members of your healthcare team to determine the screening intervention that's right for *you*.

PURPOSE OF THE HEALTH SCREEN

The periodic health examination serves multiple purposes. These visits can serve to advance the practitioner-patient relationship; to identify risk factors for future disease; to uncover current, quiescent disease; to facilitate the practitioner's decision-making; and to educate the patient.

Advance the Practitioner-Patient Relationship

In Chapter 13, I discussed the importance of forging a solid alliance between healthcare providers and healthcare consumers. In today's fast-paced world we constantly struggle to maintain the human elements in our various relationships. Like other crucial relationships, the doctor-patient relationship seems to be on the precipice of extinction!

The periodic health evaluation is usually performed when the patient is healthy, a time when both parties are not burdened with the challenges of combating an injury or illness. Therefore, the interaction is relatively more positive and facilitates the connectivity between doctor and patient.

Identify Risk Factors for Future Disease

A fundamental purpose of the periodic health visit is to identify risk factors that can predict future diseases and to identify current conditions that have not yet produced symptoms. For example, elevated low-density cholesterol (LDL or so-called "bad cholesterol") and homocysteine levels, predicts the risk for coronary heart disease and stroke in most people.

On the other hand, not finding any risk factors serves an important purpose to reinforce current lifestyle choices. A large number of people worry about having health conditions that have not yet manifested. The litany of news stories of extreme examples of diseases further fuel the fire of worry. A normal health assessment can effectively mitigate these worries.

Uncover Current, Quiescent Disease

There are a number of conditions that produce little or no symptoms and manifest themselves only after they have created significant damage. One such example is high blood pressure (dubbed "the silent killer") that is notorious for being asymptomatic until it causes a stroke, heart attack or kidney damage. This condition can easily be identified during the periodic health evaluation and promptly treated. In fact, high blood pressure is one of the most common, quiescent diseases uncovered during the periodic health evaluation. And it's one of the easiest chronic diseases to treat!

Facilitate the Practitioner's Decision-making

Doctors and other health professionals make better decisions when they are not hurried and when they're not operating under the pressure of making an emergent diagnosis. For example, being seen in a typical 15-minute appointment slot for a sick visit to evaluate the complaint of *fatigue* is very different from a 15-minute routine visit for a *general check-up*. When the practitioner doesn't feel pressured, the patient feels more relaxed and both parties reap the benefit.

Patient Education

During the general check-up, patients are typically more relaxed than when they are sick and more receptive to being educated about the need for behavioral changes and the avoidance of environmental exposures. Even when a non-acute medical condition (e.g., high blood pressure) is identified, this setting fosters a better understanding of the practitioner's explanation.

WHAT TO EXPECT DURING THE HEALTH SCREEN

In this section, I'll help you to understand the evidence-based medical recommendations of various authorities. These recommendations drive the practice style of doctors and other health workers. I'll also briefly walk you through a typical medical check-up process: the history, physical examination, laboratory and X-ray studies and medical procedures. Some providers practice differently, so your experience may vary.

Current Recommendations

As I discussed earlier, a number of governmental, patient advocacy and medical specialty organizations have position papers that spell out their recommendations for periodic health screenings for healthy people. In Appendix II, I list the contact information of most of the major health advocacy organizations such as the American Cancer Society and the American Heart Association. These recommendations are based on the organization's best judgment given the current scientific evidence.

The following Table lists the recommendation of the USPSTF for clinical preventive services for healthy women at average risk:[2]

Table 14-1

Intervention	18-35 years	40-50 years	60+ years
Immunization			
Tetanus-diphtheria (every 10 years)			X
Varicella (2 doses if none as a child)	X	X	X
Measles, mumps, rubella (1 dose)	X	X	X
Pneumococcal (one dose)	X	X	X
Influenza (yearly)			X
Screening			
Blood pressure, height, weight, dental		X	X
Alcohol use		X	X
Pap smear (every 1-3 years)	X	X	X
Cholesterol (every 5 years)	X	X	X
Mammography (every 1-2 years)	X	X	X
Sigmoidoscopy (every 5-10 years)			X
Fecal occult blood (every year)			X
Vision and hearing (periodically)		X	X
Counseling			
Calcium intake	X	X	X
Folic acid	X	X	
Hormone replacement therapy		X	X
Mammography screening		X	X
Tobacco, drugs, alcohol, sexually transmitted diseases & safety	X	X	X

History

As with all parts of the health evaluation, the health history is very important. Some doctors feel that the history is the *most* important part of the health evaluation as it paints a health picture of the patient, his or her family and provides clues to potential trouble ahead.

Physical Examination

Vital Signs. Taking the vital signs—height, weight, blood pressure, pulse, respiratory rate and temperature—is a standard part of nearly all medical office visits. Information gleaned from these parameters gives a picture of overall health. For example, an elevated blood pressure offers a glimpse of a person's cardiovascular health. An elevated pulse can be one piece of the puzzle in an attempt to rule out thyroid disease.

Eye Examination. The vision check evaluates visual acuity and uncovers such problems as near-sightedness and far-sightedness. Other conditions that can be diagnosed during the eye exam include glaucoma and high blood pressure. Persons with a family history of glaucoma and hypertension are especially prone to these conditions. We are all at risk for near- and far-sightedness, especially as we get older.

Dental Examination. This evaluation is usually done by a dentist. The doctor looks for signs of gum disease, tooth decay, and oral cancer. Everyone's at risk for these problems but tobacco users and persons with poor oral hygiene are at especially high risk. Studies are strongly connecting the dots between dental disease and heart disease, stroke, and other conditions. A set of dental X-rays are usually done to rule out cavities that are not discernable with the naked eye.

General Physical Examination. During the head, ears, nose and throat exam, the examiner observes for deviation from normal. For example, eardrum scarring might indicate previous ear infections and predict future hearing difficulty. In the neck, the lymph nodes and thyroid are palpated to detect enlargement, tenderness, and other abnormalities.

Evaluation of the heart involves looking, listening with a stethoscope, and palpating the chest wall. Murmurs, bruits, clicks and other abnormal sounds diagnose a variety of conditions. Listening to lung sounds and tapping on the chest wall help the doctor to rule out infection, masses, and other conditions in the lungs and chest cavity.

The abdomen has numerous organs such as the stomach, spleen, pancreas and liver. The provider typically employs listening, palpating, and tapping to evaluate these organs.

The musculoskeletal examination evaluates mainly the upper and lower extremities. The arms and legs are evaluated for their range of motion, strength, symmetry, and presence or absence of swelling, among other things.

Laboratory Studies

Given the high prevalence of coronary heart disease and stroke among Americans, most health advocates recommend that healthy adults undergo a lipid profile study, which involves testing for: total cholesterol; LDL cholesterol (so-called "bad cholesterol); HDL cholesterol (so-called "good cholesterol") and triglycerides.

Other commonly ordered laboratory studies include urinalysis, complete blood count, a thyroid study, fasting blood glucose, and liver and kidney studies. The recommended laboratory tests will depend on your particular health profile.

Radiographic Studies

Currently, the mammography (X-rays of the breasts) and dual-energy X-ray absorptiometry (DEXA) scan, which is an X-ray study to quantify bone mineral density (BMD), which indicates the presence or absence of osteoporosis.

DEXA Scan. As you may know, osteoporosis—thinning of the bones which leaves them prone to fractures—is at epidemic levels, affecting as estimated 44 million women and men over the age of fifty. Risk factors include being: small and thin; of older age; female gender; a smoker; a person who consumes lots of alcohol; having a diet low in calcium; and a lack of vitamin D consumption or production.

The National Osteoporosis Foundation recommends that women undergo a BMD test if they:

- Are postmenopausal and under age 65 with one or more risk factors for osteoporosis
- Are age 65 or older without any risk factors for osteoporosis
- Are postmenopausal and stopped taking estrogen therapy or hormone therapy
- Have a history of a broken bone after age 50

The best way to assess BMD is via DEXA scan, which uses two different X-ray beams to estimate BMD in the hip and spine. Dense bones allow less of the X-ray beam to penetrate through them; thin bones allow more of the X-ray beam to pass through them. The BMD is estimated based on the penetration value of the X-ray beam.

Mammogram. A mammogram is an X-ray study of the breasts. It is done to screen for breast disease in women who don't have symptoms of breast disease. It's also used to evaluate breast symptoms such as lumps, nipple discharge and color changes.

As you may know, breast cancer is the most common cancer among American women, with an estimated 182,000 new cases diagnosed each year. It's the second leading cause of cancer deaths among women, after lung cancer. The chance of a woman developing breast cancer in a lifetime is 1 in 8 (assuming a life expectancy of 80 years)!

The American Cancer Society recommends that women age 40 and older undergo a screening mammogram annually for as long as they are healthy.[3] During the exam, each breast is pressed between two plates to flatten and spread the breast tissue for better visualization. Low-level X-rays are then used to image the breasts. The most commonly reported side effect of mammography is the brief discomfort felt during compression of the breasts. The level of radiation used in this study is relatively low.

Procedures

The most common procedures associated with the periodic health evaluation of women are immunizations, the Papanicolaou (or pap) smear, flexible sigmoidoscopy, and colonoscopy.

Immunizations. One of the most controversial preventive health strategies is immunization against chronic diseases. Immunization practice represents one of the most successful public health strategies in human history. In fact, prior to widespread immunization, smallpox killed over 300 million people around the globe in the 20th century alone. Remarkably, the smallpox vaccine eradicated this public health scrooge off the face of the earth!

More recently, since the introduction of the Haemophilus influenza type B (Hib) vaccine in 1987, the incidence of Hib-induced infections, such as childhood ear infections, have decreased by more than 95 percent—undoubtedly, a major public health success story!

On the other hand, immunizations have been blamed for the recent epidemic of autism among America's children. Critics blame the mercury in the vaccine for novel genetic mutation in victims predisposed to this tragic disease. They point to the almost non-existent rates of autism among unvaccinated, homeschooled children as evidence implicating mercury in the development of autism.

Adult immunizations are less implicated in long-term disease. Finally, remember that no immunization is 100 percent effective or 100 percent safe!

Papanicolaou (Pap) Smear. The Pap smear is a non-invasive procedure done to obtain samples of cells of the uterine cervix in order to determine the health of the cervix and to rule out the presence of pre-cancer and cancer cells.

Flexible Sigmoidoscopy. This evaluation of the lower part of the colon allows the examiner to see the insides of the lower bowel. It helps determine the presence or absence of inflammation, bleeding, and abnormal growths (e.g., cancer).

Prior to the examination, you'll be given instructions to empty the contents of your bowel. Usually, patients are asked to adhere to a clear-liquid diet for 12 to 14 hours, consuming, for example, soups, strained fruit juices, water and tea. The night before the procedure, you might be asked to use an enema to thoroughly clean out the bowel.

For the procedure you'll lie on your left side on the examining table while the doctor inserts a flexible scope in your rectum with a light at its end. While advancing the scope, the doctor might blow air into the rectum. The special scope also allows the physician to biopsy any suspicious lesions for pathological analysis.

A flexible Sigmoidoscopy typically takes about 20 minutes to complete. Side effects include pressure and cramping in the lower abdomen. Risks include perforation of the bowel and bleeding, although these complications are rare.

Colonoscopy. Like a flexible Sigmoidoscopy, a colonoscopy allows the operator to visualize the inside of the bowel. However, unlike a flexible Sigmoidoscopy, a colonoscopy visualizes the entire colon. This helps determine the presence or absence of inflammation, bleeding, and abnormal growths (e.g., cancer).

Prior to the examination, you'll be given instructions to empty the contents of your bowel. Usually, patients are asked to adhere to a clear-liquid diet for 1 to 3 days, consuming, for example, soups, strained fruit juices, water and tea. The night before the procedure, you might be asked to use an enema to thoroughly clean out the bowel.

Before the procedure, you'll be given a pain medicine and a sedative to help you to relax. For the procedure you'll lie on your left side on the examining table while the doctor inserts a long, flexible scope with a light at its end into your rectum. While advancing the scope the doctor might blow air into the rectum. The special scope also allows the physician to biopsy any suspicious lesions for pathological analysis.

A colonoscopy typically takes about 30 to 60 minutes to complete. You'll need to stay in the medical facility for 1 to 2 hours after the procedure to allow the sedative to wear off. Side effects of the procedure include pressure and cramping in the lower abdomen. Risks include perforation of the bowel and bleeding, although these complications are rare.

OPTIMIZE YOUR WELLNESS VISIT

In Chapter 13, I discussed strategies for developing solid relationships with your healthcare providers. These strategies are worth repeating. A good practitioner-patient relationship is the foundation for optimizing your healthcare visit. Here are four ways to get the most out of your visit to the doctor:

Submit Your Health History & Questions Before Your Visit

A common complaint of patients is leaving their doctors' offices more confused than when they arrived! Invariably, their confusion is due to the short duration of the visit; difficulty understanding medical jargon; and reluctance to question the doctor. Submitting your health history and your questions to your doctor (via the nurse, if this is more appropriate) before the day of your visit can help eliminate confusion. Don't worry if your questions sound silly to you; if they're important enough to be asked, they're important enough for your doctor to answer them.

The health history will help the practitioner zero in on the most important aspects of your health. With your questions in front of him or her, the doctor can better target his or her discussion. If your questions are not completely answered, speak up—ask the doctor to explain his or her answer in simpler or different terms.

Be Prepared to Be a Co-partner

Many health experts believe that both the care provider and the patient should share responsibility for weighing risks and benefits when deciding on diagnostic testing and interventions. Patients generally need to be educated by the provider before they can be effective co-partners—they need good informed consent.

It might be helpful to read up on the health conditions that concern you prior to your visit. This will give you a basic understanding before the doctor's explanation.

Take Written Notes During the Visit

Typically, multiple recommendations are made during a doctor's visit. Sometimes, the recommendations are technical in nature. Writing down each recommendation and additional notes will help you to better assimilate the information flow. Your written notes can also serve as a roadmap as you implement each recommendation.

Alternatively, you can ask your provider for printed materials on the subjects discussed. Knowing that you'll be given written instructions can improve your learning as you'll not have to focus on writing new information during the healthcare visit.

Schedule a Follow-up Visit

If your doctor identifies a problem and makes recommendations for fixing the problem, it's best to make a return visit to determine if your efforts succeeded in fixing the problem. Oftentimes, a follow-up laboratory or radiographic study is needed to make this determination.

IN SUMMARY

- The periodic health assessment of the apparently healthy adult has a long history that dates back to the 1920s.
- Clinicians began questioning the value of these visits as healthcare costs began rising in the 1970s.
- Today, recommendations for the periodic physical and targeted testing are made by numerous advocate organizations including the Canadian Task Force on the Periodic Examination (CTFPHE) and the United States Preventive Services Task Force (USPSTF).
- Most advocates agree that periodic health visits can serve to advance the practitioner-patient relationship; to indentify risk factors for future disease; to uncover current, quiescent disease; to facilitate the practitioner's decision-making; and to educate the patient.
- The periodic health evaluation involves: a thorough personal and family medical history; a head-to-toe physical examination; targeted laboratory and radiographic studies (e.g., cholesterol testing and mammogram); and selected procedures (e.g., pap smear and flexible sigmoidoscopy).
- Strategies for maximizing your health visit include: Submitting your health history and your questions to your doctor (via the nurse, if this is more appropriate) before the day of your visit; reading up on the health conditions that concern you prior to your visit; taking notes during the visit; and making a follow-up visit to ensure improvement in your health.

Chapter 15

Periodic Health Assessments for Men

Preventive services for the early detection of disease have also been associated with dramatic reductions in morbidity and mortality.
—Statement in a report from Centers for Disease Control and Prevention

As I mentioned in Chapter 14, the American Medical Association (AMA), in the 1920s, recommended annual health screenings for healthy adults. Prior to that, people went to the doctor only when they were sick or injured. It was becoming clear that identifying risk factors and diseases in their early, more treatable stages was cheaper and prevented more long-term complications and deaths. However, while the AMA's intentions were noble, the extent of the annual check-up was never fully defined.

The practice of the annual health examination fell into disrepute as the cost of healthcare began to climb in the 1970s. Clinicians began questioning the return on investment as the majority of these evaluations turned up relatively little pathology (at that time). In Japan, where health promotion and disease prevention are the primary goals of the healthcare system, a relatively normal evaluation serves to reinforce good health habits, and that the *healthcare* system is doing its job to keep citizens healthy. In the US, a normal health evaluation is considered by "disease-fighters"—members of our current *sickcare* system—to be a waste of money.

In the 1970s the Canadian Task Force on the Periodic Examination (CTFPHE) was formed to evaluate the wisdom of the periodic health examination and to make recommendations for future health check-ups. In 1984, the United States Preventive Services Task Force

(USPSTF) was formed with mandates similar to its Canadian counterpart. Today, both task forces serve vital roles in helping define the periodic health examination—the CTFPHE for a true *healthcare* system and the USPSTF for a true *sickcare* system.

In addition to the CTFPHE and the USPSTF, public health agencies, patient advocacy groups and medical specialty organizations such as the American Academy of Family Physicians and the American Urological Association promulgate position papers that spell out their recommendations for periodic health screenings for apparently healthy people. A 2007 study found widespread value of the periodic health evaluation.[1]

In this Chapter, I'll synthesize the current recommendations of various advocate organizations for screening apparently healthy adult men. Because each patient is unique with his own needs, I strongly recommend that you consult your doctor and other members of your healthcare team to determine the screening intervention that's right for *you*.

PURPOSE OF THE HEALTH SCREEN

It's well-known in medical circles that American men characteristically procrastinate when it comes to seeking healthcare. Even when symptoms are present, men find ways to rationalize them away! Indeed, it's common for men to wait until they absolutely have to visit the doctor—when their symptoms (most commonly, pain) are so disabling they have no other choice.

When it comes to preventive health evaluation, men have an even more dismal track record. Surveys show that men commonly fail to get simple screenings such as blood pressure, weight, and vision checks—it's not the macho thing to do! The only way to get men to undergo periodic health check-ups is to enlist the help of their spouses or significant other.

The periodic health examination serves multiple purposes. These visits can serve to advance the practitioner-patient relationship; to indentify risk factors for future disease; identify current, quiescent disease; to facilitate the practitioner's decision-making; and to educate the patient.

Advance the Practitioner-Patient Relationship

In Chapter 13, I discussed the importance of forging a solid alliance between healthcare providers and healthcare consumers. In today's fast-paced world we constantly struggle to maintain the human elements in our various relationships. Like other crucial relationships, the doctor-patient relationship seems to be on the precipice of extinction!

The periodic health evaluation is usually performed when the patient is healthy, a time when both parties are not burdened with the challenges of injury or illness. Therefore, the interaction is relatively more positive and facilitates the connectivity between doctor and patient.

Identify Risk Factors for Future Disease

A fundamental purpose of the periodic health visit is to identify risk factors that can predict future diseases and to identify current conditions that have not yet produced symptoms. For example, elevated low-density cholesterol (LDL or so-called "bad cholesterol") and homocysteine levels, predicts the risk for coronary heart disease and stroke in most people.

Uncover Current, Quiescent Disease

There are a number of conditions that produce little or no symptoms and manifest themselves only after they have created significant damage. One such example is high blood pressure (dubbed "the silent killer") that is notorious for being asymptomatic until it causes a stroke, heart attack or kidney damage. This condition can easily be identified during the periodic health evaluation and promptly treated. In fact, high blood pressure is one of the most common, quiescent diseases uncovered during the periodic health evaluation. And it's one of the easiest chronic diseases to treat!

Facilitate the Practitioner's Decision-making

Doctors and other health professionals make better decisions when they are not hurried and when they're not operating under the pressure of making an emergent diagnosis. For example, being seen in a typical 15-minute appointment slot for a sick visit to evaluate the complaint of *fatigue* is very different from a 15-minute routine visit for a *general check-up*. When the practitioner doesn't feel pressured, the patient feels more relaxed and both parties reap the benefit.

Patient Education

During the general check-up, patients are typically more relaxed than when they are sick and more receptive to being educated about the need for behavioral changes and the avoidance of environmental exposures. Even when a non-acute medical condition (e.g., high blood pressure) is identified, this setting fosters a better understanding of the practitioner's explanation.

WHAT TO EXPECT DURING THE HEALTH SCREEN

In this section, I'll help you to understand the evidence-based medical recommendations of various authorities. These recommendations drive the practice style of doctors and other health workers. I'll also briefly walk you through a typical medical check-up process: the health history, physical examination, laboratory and X-ray studies and medical procedures. Some providers practice differently, so your experience may vary.

Current Recommendations

As I discussed earlier, a number of governmental, patient advocacy and medical specialty organizations have position papers that spell out their recommendations for periodic health screenings for healthy people. In Appendix II, I list the contact information of most of the major health advocacy organizations such as the American Cancer Society and the American Heart Association. These recommendations are based on the organization's best judgment given the current scientific evidence.

The following Table lists the recommendation of the USPSTF for clinical preventive services for healthy men at average risk:[2]

Table 15-1

Intervention	18-35 years	40-50 years	60+ years
Immunization			
Tetanus-diphtheria (every 10 years)	X	X	X
Varicella (2 doses if none as a child)	X	X	X
Pneumococcal (one dose)			X
Influenza (yearly)			X
Screening			
Blood pressure, height, weight, dental		X	X
Alcohol use		X	X
Cholesterol (every 5 years)	X	X	X
Sigmoidoscopy (every 5-10 years)	X	X	X
Fecal occult blood (every year)			X
Vision and hearing (periodically)		X	X
Counseling			
Prostate cancer screening		X	X
Tobacco, drugs, alcohol, sexually transmitted diseases & safety	X	X	X

Health History

As with all parts of the medical evaluation, the health history is very important. Some doctors feel that the history is the *most* important part of the health evaluation as it paints a health picture of the patient, his or her family and provides clues to potential trouble in the future.

Physical Examination

Vital Signs. Taking the vital signs—height, weight, blood pressure, pulse, respiratory rate and temperature—is a standard part of nearly all medical office visits. Information gleaned from these parameters gives a picture of overall health. For example, an elevated blood pressure offers a glimpse of a person's cardiovascular health. An elevated temperature when you are not ill can indicate a revved up thyroid gland.

Eye Examination. The vision check evaluates visual acuity and can uncover such problems as near-sightedness and far-sightedness. Other conditions that can be diagnosed during the eye exam include glaucoma and high blood pressure. Persons with a family history of glaucoma and hypertension are especially prone to these conditions. As we get older, we are all at risk for near- and far-sightedness.

Dental Examination. This evaluation is usually done by a dentist. The doctor looks for signs of gum disease, tooth decay, and oral cancer. Everyone's at risk for these problems but tobacco users and persons with poor oral hygiene are at especially high risk. Studies are strongly connecting the dots between dental disease and heart disease, stroke, and other conditions. A set of dental X-rays are usually done to rule out cavities that are not discernable with the naked eye.

General Physical Examination. During the head, ears, nose and throat exam, the examiner looks for deviation from normal. For example, eardrum scarring might indicate previous ear infections and predict future hearing difficulty. In the neck, the lymph nodes and thyroid gland are palpated to detect enlargement, tenderness, and other abnormalities.

Evaluation of the heart involves looking at the chest, listening with a stethoscope, and palpating the chest wall. Murmurs, bruits, clicks and other abnormal sounds diagnose a variety of conditions. Listening to lung sounds and tapping or percussing the chest wall helps the doctor to rule out infection, masses, and other conditions in the lungs and chest cavity.

The abdomen has numerous organs such as the stomach, spleen, pancreas and liver. The provider typically employs listening, palpating, and tapping to evaluate these organs.

The musculoskeletal examination evaluates mainly the upper and lower extremities. The arms and legs are evaluated for their range of motion, strength, symmetry, and presence or absence of swelling, among other things.

Laboratory Studies

Given the high prevalence of coronary heart disease and stroke among Americans, most health advocates recommend that healthy adults undergo a lipid profile study, which involves testing for: total cholesterol; LDL cholesterol (so-called "bad cholesterol"); HDL cholesterol (so-called "good cholesterol") and triglycerides.

Other commonly ordered laboratory studies include urinalysis, complete blood count, a thyroid study, fasting blood glucose, and liver and kidney studies. The recommended laboratory tests will depend on your particular health profile.

Radiographic Studies

Currently, no organization recommends routine radiographic studies for the apparently healthy adult. The only X-ray study recommended as a screening tool is the bone mineral density (BMD) done to evaluate bone health, which screens for osteoporosis. As you may know, osteoporosis—thinning of the bones which leaves them prone to fractures—is at epidemic levels, affecting as estimated 44 million women and men over the age of fifty. Risk factors include being: small and thin; older age; a smoker; a person who consumes lots of alcohol; and having a diet low in calcium; and a lack of vitamin D. Men are at lower risk than are women.

The National Osteoporosis Foundation recommends that men undergo a BMD test if they:

- Are age 50-70 with one or more risk factors for osteoporosis
- Are age 70 or older without any risk factors for osteoporosis
- Have a history of broken bone after age 50

The most common way to assess BMD is via the dual-energy X-ray absorptiometry (DEXA) scan. DEXA uses two different X-ray beams to estimate BMD in the hip and spine. Dense bones allow less of the X-ray beam to penetrate through them; thin bones allow more of the X-ray beam to pass through them. The BMD is estimated based on the penetration value of the X-ray beam.

Procedures

The most common procedures associated with the periodic health evaluation of men are immunizations, the digital rectal examination of the prostate, flexible sigmoidoscopy, and colonoscopy.

Immunizations. One of the most controversial preventive health strategies is immunization against chronic diseases. Immunization practice represents one of the most successful public health strategies in human history. For example, prior to widespread immunization, smallpox killed over 300 million people around the globe in the 20th century alone. Remarkably, the smallpox vaccine eradicated this public health scrooge off the face of the earth!

More recently, since the introduction of the Haemophilus influenza type B (Hib) vaccine in 1987, the incidence of Hib-induced infections, such as childhood ear infections, have decreased by more than 95 percent—undoubtedly, a major public health success story!

On the other hand, immunizations have been blamed for the recent epidemic of autism among America's children. Critics blame the mercury in the vaccine for novel genetic mutation in victims predisposed to this tragic disease. They point to the almost non-existent rates of autism among unvaccinated, homeschooled children as evidence implicating mercury in the development of autism.

Adult immunizations are less implicated in long-term disease. Remember that no immunization is 100 percent effective or 100 percent safe!

Digital Rectal Examination. The digital rectal examination is a non-invasive procedure done to palpate the prostate gland in order to rule out asymmetry, lumps, tenderness, and other abnormalities. Prostate cancer is at epidemic proportions among older American men.

Flexible Sigmoidoscopy. This evaluation of the lower part of the colon allows the examiner to see the insides of the lower bowel. This helps determine the presence or absence of inflammation, bleeding, and abnormal growths (e.g., cancer).

Prior to the examination, you'll be given instructions to empty the contents of your bowel. Usually, patients are asked to adhere to a clear-liquid diet for 12 to 14 hours, consuming, for example, soups, strained fruit juices, water and tea. The night before the procedure, you might be asked to use an enema to thoroughly clean out the bowel.

For the procedure you'll lie on your left side on the examining table while the doctor inserts a flexible scope into your rectum with a light at its end. While advancing the scope, the doctor might blow air into the rectum. The special scope also allows the physician to biopsy any suspicious lesions for pathological analysis.

A flexible Sigmoidoscopy typically takes about 20 minutes to complete. Side effects include pressure and cramping in the lower abdomen.

Risks include perforation of the bowel and bleeding, although these complications are rare.

Colonoscopy. Like a flexible Sigmoidoscopy, a colonoscopy allows the operator to visualize the inside of the bowel. However, unlike a flexible Sigmoidoscopy, a colonoscopy visualizes the entire colon. This helps determine the presence or absence of inflammation, bleeding, and abnormal growths (e.g., cancer).

Prior to the examination, you'll be given instructions to empty the contents of your bowel. Usually, patients are asked to adhere to a clear-liquid diet for 1 to 3 days, consuming, for example, soups, strained fruit juices, water and tea. The night before the procedure, you might be asked to use an enema to thoroughly clean out the bowel.

Before the procedure, you'll be given a pain medicine and a sedative to help you to relax. For the procedure you'll lie on your left side on the examining table while the doctor inserts a long, flexible scope with a light at its end into your rectum. While advancing the scope the doctor might blow air into the rectum. The special scope also allows the physician to biopsy any suspicious lesions for pathological analysis.

A colonoscopy typically takes about 30 to 60 minutes to complete. You'll need to stay in the medical facility for 1 to 2 hours after the procedure to allow the sedative to wear off. Side effects of the procedure include pressure and cramping in the lower abdomen. Risks include perforation of the bowel and bleeding, although these complications are rare.

OPTIMIZE YOUR WELLNESS VISIT

In Chapter 13, I discussed strategies for developing solid relationships with your healthcare team. Those strategies are worth repeating. A good practitioner-patient relationship is the foundation for optimizing your healthcare visit. Here are four ways to get the most out of your visit to the doctor:

Submit Your Health History & Questions Before Your Visit

A common complaint of patients is leaving their doctors' offices more confused than when they arrived! Invariably, their confusion is due to the short duration of the visit; difficulty understanding medical jargon; and reluctance to question the doctor. Submitting your health history and your questions to your doctor (via the nurse, if this is more appropriate) before the day of your visit can help eliminate confusion. Don't worry if your questions sound silly to you; if they're important enough to be asked, they're important enough for your doctor to answer them.

The health history will help the practitioner zero in on the most important aspects of your health. With your questions in front of him or her, the doctor can better target his or her discussion. If your questions are not completely answered, speak up—ask the doctor to explain his or her answer in simpler or different terms.

Be Prepared to Be a Co-partner

As I discuss in Chapter 13, many experts believe that both the care provider and the patient should share responsibility for weighing risks and benefits when deciding on diagnostic testing and interventions. Patients generally need to be educated by the provider before they can be effective co-partners—they need good informed consent.

It might be helpful to read up on the health conditions that concern you prior to your visit. This will give you a basic understanding before the doctor's explanation.

Take Written Notes During the Visit

Typically, multiple recommendations are made during a doctor's visit. Sometimes, the recommendations are technical in nature. Writing down each recommendation and additional notes will help you to better assimilate the information flow. Your written notes can also serve as a roadmap as you implement each recommendation.

Alternatively, you can ask your provider for printed materials on the subjects discussed. Knowing that you'll be given written instructions can improve your learning as you'll not have to focus on writing new information during the healthcare visit.

Schedule a Follow-up Visit

If your doctor identifies a problem and makes recommendations for fixing the problem, it's best to make a return visit to determine if your efforts succeeded in fixing the problem. Oftentimes, a follow-up laboratory or radiographic study is needed to make this determination.

IN SUMMARY

- The periodic health assessment of the apparently healthy adult has a long history that dates back to the 1920s.
- Clinicians began questioning the value of these visits as healthcare costs began rising in the 1970s.
- Today, recommendations for the periodic physical and targeted testing are made by numerous advocate organizations including the Canadian Task Force on the Periodic Examination (CTFPHE) and the United States Preventive Services Task Force (USPSTF).
- Most advocates agree that periodic health visits can serve to advance the practitioner-patient relationship; to indentify risk factors for future disease; to uncover current, quiescent disease; to facilitate the practitioner's decision-making; and to educate the patient.
- The periodic health evaluation involves: a thorough personal and family medical history; a head-to-toe physical examination;

targeted laboratory and radiographic studies (e.g., cholesterol testing and DEXA scan); and selected procedures (e.g., digital rectal exam and flexible sigmoidoscopy).

- Strategies for maximizing your health visit include: Submitting your health history and your questions to your doctor (via the nurse, if this is more appropriate) before the day of your visit; reading up on the health conditions that concern you prior to your visit; taking notes during the visit; and making a follow-up visit to ensure improvement in your health.

Chapter 16

Other Wellness Strategies

"I drive way too fast to worry about cholesterol."
—Author Unknown

A number of other time-honored strategies can help keep you healthy and well. These include: limiting your sun exposure; wearing seatbelts when in a vehicle; wearing protective headgear when skiing, riding a motorcycle or bicycle, wrestling, boxing and other sports involving trauma to the head; and minimizing the use of cell phones.

LIMIT SUN EXPOSURE

Most cases of skin cancer are caused by ultraviolet radiation, commonly from the sun.[1] Individuals with fair complexion are at higher risk for skin cancer than people with darker skin. Limiting outdoor activities between the hours of 10:00 am and 4:00 pm can reduce your risk.

When outside activities are warranted during the day, you should wear sunscreen. But sunscreen appears to be a double-edge sword! Experts estimate that a SPF 15 can reduce the body's natural vitamin D production by 95 percent, which can negatively impact bone health (see Chapter 3) and leave a person susceptible to skin cancer.

Another important strategy for beating skin cancer (through early detecting) is annual skin examinations by a dermatologist or family health practitioner. The best time to get your skin checked is the middle of winter when you tend to be less tanned and likely to create a bigger contrast between your skin and a suspicious lesion (that are usually pigmented). However, don't wait until your tan is gone to report suspicious lesions to your doctor.

WEAR SEATBELTS

"Seatbelts save lives" is more than a cute slogan; it's one of the best strategies for preventing physical injuries and death if involved in a motor vehicle accident. A litany of scientific and anecdotal evidence bears this out, and all States have enacted laws mandating seatbelts for motor vehicle occupants.[2] Nevertheless, many people resist buckling up and pay the price with their lives!

WEAR PROTECTIVE HEAD GEAR

The brain is one of the most vulnerable organs in the body. Protecting it is a crucial health promotion and disease prevention strategy.[3] I recommend that you wear protective gear for your given sport or recreational activity. Skiing is fun and healthy but it would be sad if your fun is cut short by a preventable head injury.

Riding a bicycle is one of the healthiest physical activities around. However, this very healthy activity can quickly turn into a nightmare if you are hit by a vehicle or if you fall off your bike and hit your head. One of the most common injuries sustained in motor cycle accidents is head injury. Wearing an approved helmet can be the difference between a non-life-threatening and a life-threatening accident. Please pay heed!

MINIMIZE CELL PHONE USAGE

Cell phone use has come under scrutiny in recent years due to their use during driving and the risk for auto accidents. More recently, neurologist Dr. David Perlmutter of the Perlmutter Health Center and other prominent brain health specialists are sounding the cry for limiting cell phone usage due to possible adverse health effects.[4] They fear that prolonged radiation levels and electromagnetic energy generated within close proximity of the brain might be bad for brain health. That there's been a dramatic rise in brain tumors in the past decade can probably be traced to the escalating use of cell phones. Experts recommend using a hands-free device to minimize direct exposure of the brain to electromagnetic radiation.

IN SUMMARY

- Limiting exposure to the sun by minimizing outdoor activities and wearing sunscreen when outside are two important ways to reduce your chances of developing skin cancer. Additionally, annual skin examinations (during the winter months) by a dermatologist or family physician can improve the chances of finding skin cancer early.
- Seatbelts save lives is more than a cute slogan; it is one of the best strategies for preventing physical injuries and premature death.
- Motorcycle and bicycle helmets help prevent one of the most common injuries during a bicycle accident—fatal head injuries. Study after study concludes that wearing a helmet while riding a motorcycle or bicycle is a good way to help stay alive and well.

Chapter 17

Epilogue

"The best six doctors anywhere
And no one can deny it
Are sunshine, water rest and air
Exercise and diet
These six will gladly you attend
If only you are willing
Your mind they'll ease
Your will they'll mend
And charge you not a shilling."
—Nursery Rhyme quoted by Wayne Fields
What the River Knows, 1990

I hope that *Prescription for Wellness* came close to fulfilling its intended goal: to serve as a single source, self-help manual to help you achieve optimal health, wellness and longevity under the advisement of your physician or other health professional. I articulated for you the scientific evidence, accumulated over the past four-plus decades, which unequivocally reveals that lifestyle choices trump genetic endowment when it comes to the development of chronic diseases and how long you live.

The next step is up to you. The ball is in your court. Only *you* can decide to:

- Eat healthfully
- Take selected supplements, if needed
- Accumulate at least 60 minutes (or 10,000 steps) of physical activity each day

- Achieve a BMI that's healthy for your height
- Adhere to proven strategies that can help you get at least 7 hours of restful sleep each night
- Manage your stress strategically
- Stop using cigarettes, cigars or smokeless tobacco products
- Drink alcohol in moderate amounts, if at all
- Weave a solid network of relationships with friends and relatives
- Develop solid relationships with your healthcare team
- Go for periodic health assessments as recommended by your doctor
- Limit your sun exposure
- Wear seatbelts
- Wear protective headgear
- Minimize cell phone usage

DEVELOP A COMPREHENSIVE PLAN

I suggest that you sit down with your primary care provider and let him or her know what you've learned in this book. If cleared to do so by your doctor, ask him or her to help you develop a Wellness Life Plan, then start implementing what you've learned. Be sure to ask your doctor to discuss which symptoms (e.g., chest pains, lightheadedness, etc) you should consider urgent or emergent and what to do if these symptoms occur while implementing your plan.

If you currently have many healthy habits to adopt, I'd recommend you do so slowly and incrementally all the while keeping your healthcare provider apprised of your progress.

PUTTING IT ALL TOGETHER

I've presented you a lot of information that can be overwhelming. This book is meant to be a catalogue of strategies for a healthy lifestyle including dietary measures, exercise program, and stress management. Now it's up to you to take a proactive role in controlling your blood pressure and, hopefully, in your overall health. Good health is your most precious possession; protect it the best way you know how. You owe it to yourself and your family!

IN THE FUTURE

Where do you go from here? Scientific research and clinical observations continually provide new insight into health and wellness issues. You should stay abreast of these changes, and I'll do so as well and will incorporate any changes in future editions of this book.

In the meantime, please feel free to jot down your comments, thoughts, and suggestions regarding wellness in general and this book in particular, and send them directly to me at the following address:

Dr. Ceabert J. Griffith
205-11 Tamagami, Chatan-cho
Okinawa, Japan 904-0106
e-mail: prescriptionforwellness@yahoo.com

Please stay Well!!!!!

Notes

Introduction

1. L. Breslow, L, and J. E. Enstrom. Persistence of health habits and their relationship to mortality. *Preventive Medicine*. 9(1980):469-483.

2. R. Eberst. Defining Health: A Multidimensional Model. *Journal of School Health*. 54(1984):99-104.

Chapter 1

1. J. W. Rowe and R. L. Kahn. *Successful Aging*. New York: Pantheon: 1998.

2. B. J. Willcox, D. C. Willcox and M. Suzuki. *The Okinawa Diet Plan*. New York: Clarkson Potter: 2004.

3. D. Buettner. *The Blue Zones*. Washington, D.C: The National Geographic Society: 2008.

Chapter 2

1. M. Pollan. In Defense of Food: An Eater's Manifesto. New York, NY: Penguin Books, 2008.

2. H. Todoriki. A Clinical Trial of the Effects of the Traditional Okinawan Diet on Blood Pressure and Other Health Indicators:

Can DASH-like Results be Achieved? Presented at the 22nd Scientific Meeting of the International Society of Hypertension. June 14-19, 2008 in Berlin, Germany.

3. Os de Santos and R. A. Johns. Effects of garlic powder and garlic oil preparations on blood lipids, blood pressure and well-being. *British Journal of Clinical Research.* 6(1995):91-100.

4. F. M. Sacks, A. Lichtenstein, L. Van Horn, et al. Soy protein, isoflavones, and cardiovascular health: an American Heart Association science advisory for professionals from the nutrition committee. *Circulation.* 113(2006):1034-1044.

5. N. Katsube, K. Iwashita, T. Tsushida, et al. Induction of apoptosis in cancer cells by Bilberry (Vaccinium myrtillus) and anthocyanins. *Journal of Agricultural and Food Chemistry.* (51)2003:68-75.

6. H. Nishino, M. Murakosh, T. Li, et al. Carotenoids in cancer chemoprevention. *Cancer Metastasis Review.* 21(2002):257-264.

7. G. S. Omenn, G. E. Goodman, M. D. Thornquist, et al. Risk factors for lung cancer and for intervention effects in CARET, the beta-carotene and retinol efficacy trial. *Journal of the National Cancer Institute.* 88(1996):1550-1559.

8. S. Chen, O. Sei-Ryang, S. Phung, et al. Anti-aromatase activity of phytochemicals in white button mushrooms. *Cancer Research.* 66(2006):12026-12034.

Chapter 3

1. S. S. Casagrande, Y. Wang, C. Anderson, and T. L. Gary. Have Americans increased their fruit and vegetable intake? The trends between 1988 and 2002. *American Journal of Preventive Medicine.* (32)2007:257-263.

2. A. Weil. Healthy Aging. New York, NY: Anchor Books: 2007.

3. X. Zhao, G. Aldini, E. J. Johnson, et al. Modification of lymphocyte DNA damage by carotenoid supplementation in postmenopausal women. *American Journal of Clinical Nutrition.* 83(2006):163-169.

4. H. McNulty, G. J. Cuskelly, and M. Ward. Response of red blood cell folate to intervention: implications for folate recommendations for the prevention of neural tube defects. *American Journal of Clinical Nutrition.* 71(2000):1308S-1311S.

5. E. Giovannucci, M. J. Stampfer, G. A. Colditz, et al. Multivitamin use, folate, and colon cancer in women in the Nurses' Health Study. *Ann Intern Med.* 129(1998):517-524.

6. From the Homocysteine Lowering Trialists' Collaboration. Dose-dependent effects of folic acid on blood concentrations of homocysteine: a meta-analysis of the randomized trials. *American Journal of Clinical Nutrition.* 82(2005):806-812.

7. L. Podoshin, R. Gertner, and M. Fradis. Treatment of perennial allergic rhinitis with ascorbic acid solution. *Ear Nose and Throat Journal.* 70(1991):54-55.

8. S. Duffy, N. Gokce, M. Holbrook, et al. Treatment of hypertension with ascorbic acid. *Lancet.* 354(1999):248-249.

9. L. E. Griffith, G. H. Guyatt, R. J. Cook, et al. The influence of dietary and non-dietary calcium supplementation on blood pressure: an updated meta-analysis of randomized controlled trials. *American Journal of Hypertension.* 12(1999):84-92.

10. A. Ascherio, E. B. Rimm, E. L. Giovannucci, et al. A prospective study of nutrition factors and hypertension among US men. *Circulation.* 86(1992):1651-1653.

11. Veterans Administration Cooperative Study Group on Antihypertensive Agents. Urinary and serum electrolytes in untreated black and white hypertensives. *Journal of Chronic Diseases*. 40(1987):839-847.

12. S. Gao, Y. Jin, K. S. Hall, et al. Selenium level and cognitive function in rural elderly Chinese. *American Journal of Epidemiology*. 165(2007):955-965.

13. W-Q. Wei, C. C. Abnet, Y-L. Qiao, et al. Prospective study of serum selenium concentrations and esophageal and gastric cardia cancer, heart disease, stroke, and total death. *American Journal of Clinical Nutrition*. 79(2004):80-85.

14. L. Holmquist, G. Stuchbury, K. Berbaum, et al. Lipoic acid as a novel treatment for Alzheimer's disease and related dementias. *Pharmacological Therapeutics*. 113(2007):154-164.

15. M. J. Budoff, J. Takasu, F. R. Flores, et al. Inhibiting progression of coronary calcification using aged garlic extract in patients receiving statin therapy: a preliminary study. *Preventive Medicine*. (39)2004:985-991.

16. M. Steiner, W. Li. Aged garlic extract, a modulator of cardiovascular risk factors: a dose-finding study on the effects of AGE on platelet functions. *Journal of Nutrition*. 131(2001):980S-984S.

Chapter 4

1. T. W. Stine, A. H. Mokdad, S. R. Dube, et al. The association of depression and anxiety with obesity and unhealthy behaviors among community-dwelling US adults. *General Hospital Psychiatry*. 30(2008):127-137.

2. T. Thom, N. Hasse, W. Rosamund, et al. Heart disease and stroke statistics—2006 update. *Circulation*. 113(2006):e85-e151.

3. National Osteoporosis Foundation. www.nof.org

4. American Cancer Society. www.cancer.org

5. American College of Sports Medicine. Position Stand: Exercise and Hypertension. *Medicine and Science in Sports and Exercise.* 36(2004):533-553.

6. N. Mutrie, A. M. Campbell, F. Whyte, et al. Benefits of supervised group exercise programme for women being treated for early stage breast cancer: Pragmatic randomised controlled trial. *British Medical Journal.* 334(2007):517.

U.S. Department of Health and Human Services, Washington, D.C. *2008 Physical Activity Guidelines for Americans.* www.health.gov/paguidelines

Chapter 5

1. I-M. Lee, S. N. Blair, D. B Allison. Epidemiological data on the relationship of caloric intake, energy balance, and weight gain over the life span with longevity and morbidity. *Journal of Gerontology*. 56(2001):7-19.

2. C. A. Maglione-Garves, L. Kravitz, and S. Schneider. Cortisol connection: Tips on managing stress and weight. *Health & Fitness Journal.* 9(2005):20-23.

3. E. S. Epel, B. McEwen, S. Teresa, et al. Stress and body shape: Stress-induced cortisol secretion is consistently greater among women with central fat. *Psychosomatic Medicine*. 62(2000):623-632.

Chapter 6

1. National Sleep Foundation. 2005 Sleep in America Poll. Available at: http://www.sleepfoundation.org/_content/hottopics/2005_summary_of_findings.pdf.

2. P. J. Moore, N.E. Adler, D.R. Williams, and J. S. Jackson. Socioeconomic status and health: The role of sleep. *Psychosomatic Medicine.* 64(2002):337-344.

3. National Highway Traffic Safety Commission. Drowsy and distracted driving. Available at: http://www.nhtsa.dot.gov/portal/site/nhtsa/menuitem.

4. A. Rechtschaffen. Current perspectives on the function of sleep. *Perspectives in Biological Medicine.* 41(1998):359-390.

5. G. D. Mellinger, M. B. Balter, and E. H. Uhlenhuth. Insomnia and its treatment: prevalence and correlates. *Archives in General Psychiatry.* 42(1985):225-232.

6. D. F. Dinges, S. D. Douglas, L. Zaugg, et al. Leukocytosis and natural-killer-cell function parallel neurobehavioral fatigue induced by 64 hours of sleep deprivation. *Journal of Clinical Investigation.* 93(1994):1930-1939.

7. H. Moldofsky, F. A. Lue, J. Dickstein, et al. Disordered circadian sleep-wake neuroendocrine and immune functions in chronic fatigue syndrome. *Advances in Neuroimmunology.* 5(1999):39-56.

8. J. Ellenbogen. "*Sleep Strengthens your Memory.*" Presented at the 59th Annual Scientific Meeting of the American Academy of Neurology held May 2007, in Boston.

9. M. M. Ohayon. Prevalence of DSM-IV diagnostic criteria of insomnia: distinguishing insomnia related to mental disorders from sleep disorder. *Journal of Psychiatric Research.* 31(1997):333-346.

10. D. E. Ford, and D. B. Kamerow. Epidemiologic study of sleep disturbances and psychiatric disorders. An opportunity for prevention? *Journal of American Medical Association.* 262(1989):1479-1484.

11. D. E. Giles, D. J. Kupfer, A. J. Rush, and H. P. Roffwarg. Controlled comparison of electrophysiological sleep pattern in families of probands with unipolar depression. *American Journal of Psychiatry.* 155(1998):192-199.

12. J. E. Gangwisch, S. B. Heymsfield, B. Boden-Albala, et al. Short sleep duration as a risk factor for hypertension. *Hypertension.* 47(2006):833-839.

13. O. Tochikubo, A. Ikeda, E. Miyajima, and M. Ishii. Effects of insufficient sleep on blood pressure monitored by a new multibiomedical recorder. *Hypertension.* 27(1996):1318-1324.

14. "Lack of Sleep May Be Deadly." Reuters News, Sept 24th 2007. http://uk.reuters.com/article/healthNews/idUKL2462796020070924 Accessed December 26th 2008.

15. K. Eguchi, T.G. Pickering, et al. Short sleep duration as an independent predictor of cardiovascular events in Japanese patients with hypertension. *Archives of Internal Medicine.* 168(2008):2225-2231.

16. R. D. Verona, M. P. Winn, T. W. Babineau, et al. Overweight and obese patients in a primary care population report less sleep than patients with a normal body mass index. *Archives of Internal Medicine.* 165(2005):25-30.

17. Eva van Cauter of the University of Chicago immunized sleep-deprived students with the flu vaccine, their immune systems failed to produce the predictable number of antibodies, but they produced high levels of cortisol, a hormone associated with stress.

18. D. J. Scott, M. M. Heitzeg, R. A. Koeppe, et al. Variations in the human pain stress experience mediated by ventral and dorsal basal ganglia dopamine activity. *Journal of Neuroscience.* 26(2006):10789-10795.

19. M. Preyde. Effectiveness of massage therapy for subacute low-back pain: A randomized controlled trial. *Canadian Medical Journal.* 162(2000):1815-1820.

20. W.I. Najm, S. Reinsch, F. Hoehler, J.S. Tobis, and P.W. Harvey. S-adenosyl methionine (SAMe) versus celecoxib for the treatment of osteoarthritis symptoms: a double-blind cross-over trial. *BMC Musculoskeletal Disorder*. 5(2004):6.

21. R. Sahelian. *5-HTP: Nature's serotonin solution*. New York: Avery Books: 1998.

Chapter 7

1. E. R. Epel, B. Lapidus, B. McEwen, et al. Stress may add bite to appetite in women: a laboratory study of stress-induced cortisol and eating. *Psychoneuroendocrinology*. 26(2001):37-49.

2. "Stress." American Psychological Association. http://www.apahelpcenter.org/articles/article.php?id=11. Accessed May 10, 2007.

3. F. Cohen, M. E. Kemeny, K. A. Kearney, et al. Persistent stress as a predictor of genital herpes recurrence. *Archives of Internal Medicine*. 159(1999):2430-2436.

4. E. Mallon, J. N. Newton, and A. F. Klassen. The quality of life in acne: a comparison with general medical conditions using generic questionnaires. *British Journal of Dermatology*. 140(1999):672-676.

5. J. E. Gallacher, P. E. Sweetnam, J. W. Yarnell, et al. Is type A behavior really a trigger for coronary heart disease events? *Psychosomatic Medicine*. 65(2003):339-346.

6. R. Stamm, L. M. A. Akkermans, and V. M. Wiegant. Trauma and the gut: Interactions between stressful experience and intestinal function. *Gut*. 40(1997):704-709.

7. S. Levenstein. Stress and peptic ulcer: life beyond helicobacter. *British Medical Journal*. 316(1998):538-541.

8. C. A. Maglione-Garves, L. Kravitz, and S. Schneider. Cortisol connection: Tips on managing stress and weight. *Health & Fitness Journal.* 9(2005):20-23.

9. E. S. Epel, B. McEwen, S. Teresa, et al. Stress and body shape: Stress-induced cortisol secretion is consistently greater among women with central fat. *Psychosomatic Medicine.* 62(2000):623-632.

Chapter 8

1. L. F. Berkman. The role of social relations in health promotion. 57(1995):245-254.

2. P. Grazzziano, R. C. Agis-Balboa, D. Mohemed-Salim, et al. Brain neurosteriods in gender-related aggression induced by social isolation. Critical Reviews in Neurobiology. (16)2004:75-82.

3. E. B. Loucks, L. Sullivan, R. B. A'Agostino, et al. "*Social Connections: Could Heart Warming be Heart-Saving?*" Presented at the American Heart Association's 45th Annual Conference on Cardiovascular Disease Epidemiology and Prevention held May 2005, in Washington, DC.

4. J. G. Grzywacz and C. L. M. Keys. Toward health promotion: The net contributions of physical and social behaviors. 28(2004):99-111.

Chapter 9

1. G. Anadarjah and E. Hight. Spirituality and medical practice: Using the HOPE questions as a practical tool for spiritual assessment. *American Family Physician.* 63(201):81-89.

2. D. Buettner. *The Blue Zones.* Washington, D.C: The National Geographic Society, 2008.

Chapter 10

1. S. Sabia, M. Marmot, C Dufouil, and A. Singh-Manoux. Smoking history and cognitive function in middle-age from the Whitehall II study. *Archives of Internal Medicine.* 168(2008):1165-1173.

2. J. Thornton, R. Edwards, P. Mitchell, et al. Smoking and age-related macular degeneration: a review of association. *Eye.* 19(2005):935-944.

3. J. Stamler, D. Wentworth, and J. Neaton, for the MRFIT Research Group. The Multiple Risk Factor Intervention Trial (MRFIT). *Journal of the American Medical Association.* 256(1986):2823-2828.

4. A. R. White, H. Rampes, and J. L. Campbell. Acupuncture and related intervention for smoking cessation. *Cochrane Database System Review.* 2006 Jan 25: CD000009.

Chapter 11

1. J. A. Ewing. Detecting alcoholism: The CAGE questionnaire. *Journal of the American Medical Association.* 252(1984):1905-1907.

Chapter 12

1. M. Hyman and M. Liponis. *Ultraprevention.* New York, NY: Atria Books, 2003.

Chapter 13

1. S.R Hahn, et al. The difficult patient: prevalence, psychopathology, and functional impairment. *Journal of General Internal Medicine.* 11(1996):1-8.

2. K. M Marvel, et al. Soliciting the patient's agenda: Have we improved? *Journal of the American Medical Association.* 281(1999):283-287.

Chapter 14

1. L. E. Boulware, S. Marinopoulos, K. A. Phillips, et al. Systematic review: The value of the periodic health evaluation. *Annals of Internal Medicine*. 146(2007):289-300.

2. USPSTF. Guide to Clinical Preventive Services, 2008. Alexandria, VA. Report of the U.S. Preventive Services Task Force. International Medical Publishing, Inc.

3. American Cancer Society. www.cancer.org. Accessed December 27, 2008.

Chapter 15

1. L. E. Boulware, S. Marinopoulos, K. A. Phillips, et al. Systematic review: The value of the periodic health evaluation. *Annals of Internal Medicine*. 146(2007):289-300.

2. USPSTF. Guide to Clinical Preventive Services, 2008. Alexandria, VA. Report of the U.S. Preventive Services Task Force. International Medical Publishing, Inc.

Chapter 16

1. American Academy of Dermatology. www.aad.org. Accessed December 27, 2008.

2. M. Ichikawa, S. Nakahara, and S. Wakai. Mortality of front-seat occupants attributable to unbelted rear-seat passengers in car crashes. *Lancet*. 359(2002):43-44.

3. Brain Injury Association of America. www.biausa.org. Accessed December 72, 2008.

4. D. Perlmutter. *The Better Brain Book: The Best Tools for Improving Memory and Sharpness and Preventing Aging of the Brain*. New York: Riverhead Books: 2004.

Glossary

Adrenal glands. A pair of glands located on top of the kidneys that secret hormones, including aldosterone, cortisone, and adrenaline, that regulate blood pressure and kidney function.

Adrenaline. Also called epinephrine, adrenaline is the "fight or flight" hormone secreted by the adrenal glands (which sit atop the kidneys). It can quickly increase heart rate and blood pressure in response to emotional or physical threat.

Aerobic exercise. Vigorous physical activity that enhances the body's intake and utilization of oxygen. An important aspect of cardiovascular fitness, aerobic exercise includes jogging, running, swimming, walking, and bicycling. See also *anaerobic exercise.*

Anaerobic exercise. An exercise whose energy comes from burning fat without the use of oxygen.

Arteries. Blood vessels that carry blood away from the heart to different parts of the body.

Arterioles. Small arteries that carry the blood from the arteries to the capillaries. Narrowing of the arterioles increases resistance to blood flow, driving up blood pressure in the larger arteries.

Arteriosclerosis. Hardening of the arteries caused by, in most cases, mineral and fatty deposits, that eventually leads to blockage of blood flow in the arteries. See also *atherosclerosis.*

Atherosclerosis. The most prevalent form of arteriosclerosis, atherosclerosis involves a buildup of hard plaques (consisting of cholesterol, fat, calcium deposits, and other debris) on the inside lining of the arteries. See also *arteriosclerosis.*

Autonomic nervous system. Also referred to as the involuntary nervous system, the autonomic nervous system regulates bodily functions not under conscious control, such as blood pressure and heart beat. The autonomic nervous system consists of two divisions: the *sympathetic* system, which narrows blood vessels and increases heart rate, and the *parasympathetic* system, which dilates blood vessels and lowers heart rate.

Biofeedback. Immediate information about a bodily function (such as heart beat and blood pressure) through audiovisual feedback that allows a person to change the level of that body function through relaxation and other methods of operant conditioning.

Blood pressure. The pressure created by the circulating blood on the walls of the arteries. Blood pressure results from the contraction, or squeezing, of the heart vis-à-vis the resistance put up by the circumference of the blood vessels. Many hormones, enzymes, and blood vessel structures influence blood pressure. Blood pressure is also influenced by the volume of circulating blood.

Blood pressure cuff. The instrument used to measure the blood pressure. See *sphygmomanometer.*

Blood volume. The total amount of blood circulating in the body.

Capillaries. The smallest blood vessels that carry blood between the arterioles and the veins. Capillaries have thin walls that allow the exchange of oxygen and other vital substances and carbon dioxide and other waste products.

Cardiovascular. Relating to the heart (cardio) and the body's network of blood vessels (vascular). Thus, cardiovascular disease refers to disease of the heart and blood vessels, including arteriosclerosis.

Carotenoids. A group of compounds that are precursors of vitamin A. These compounds, which include beta-carotene and lycopene, are converted to vitamin A in the liver.

Carotid arteries. The two main arteries that supply blood to the head and neck.

Catecholamines. Powerful chemicals (including dopamine, epinephrine, and norepinephrine) produced by the body to help regulate numerous bodily processes including heart rate and blood pressure.

Cholesterol. Waxy substance produced by the body (and also found in animal fat and dairy products) that is necessary for the production of hormones and cell function.

Computerized axial tomography. Commonly referred to as CAT scan, this X-ray procedure produces a computer-enhanced picture of a cross section of the body.

Constriction. Narrowing of blood vessels cause by contraction of their muscles.

Coronary artery disease. Diseases affecting the arteries that supply blood to the heart muscle. The most common type of coronary artery disease is atherosclerosis—the deposit of fat, cholesterol, and calcium on the inner walls of the coronary arteries.

Corticosteroids. Steroid hormones secreted by the adrenal glands. There are two main groups of corticosteroids: *glucocorticoids* (e.g., cortisone), which help the body utilize carbohydrate, fat, and protein, and *mineralocorticoids* (e.g., aldosterone), which help the kidneys regulate salt and water balance.

DEXA scan. See dual-energy X-ray absorptiometry.

Dual-energy X-ray absorptiometry (DEXA) scan. DEXA uses two different X-ray beams to estimate the density of bone. Dense bones allow less of the X-ray beam to penetrate through them; thin bones allow more of the X-ray beam to pass through them. The bone density is estimated based on the penetration value of the X-ray beam. Bone density is done to rule out osteoporosis, abnormal thinning of the bone that makes it prone to fracture.

Diabetes mellitus. Commonly referred to as diabetes, this disease has to do with the body's inability to properly utilize sugars, causing too much glucose in the blood. There are two types of diabetes mellitus: in Type I the body doesn't produce enough insulin; in Type II the body produces enough insulin but is unable to use it efficiently.

Diastole. The second (relaxation) phase of the heart cycle, when the heart chamber fills in preparation for systole (contraction).

Diastolic blood pressure. The bottom number of the blood pressure. It reflects the pressure inside the arteries when the heart is relaxed between beats. If the blood pressure is 110/68 mm Hg, the diastolic pressure is 68 mm Hg.

Echocardiogram. Also called ultrasound, this test outlines the size, structure, and function of the heart and major blood vessels by using high-frequency sound waves bounced off these structures.

Electrocardiogram. Also referred to as an EKG or ECG, this test delineates the electrical activity of the heart, and can provide information regarding the heart's muscle thickness and the presence of a heart attack and other problems.

Electrolytes. Dissolved of minerals carried by the blood that are important for muscle and other vital body functions. Electrolytes include sodium, chloride, potassium, and carbon dioxide.

Endocrine system. A system of glands that manufacture hormones. Endocrine glands include the thyroid gland, the adrenal glands, the ovaries, and the testes.

Epinephrine. Also called adrenaline, this hormone has important functions in regulation of your blood pressure. See *adrenaline*.

Essential hypertension. Also called primary or idiopathic hypertension, essential hypertension is the most common form of high blood pressure, present in about 90% of persons diagnosed with hypertension.

Estrogen. One of the female sex hormones that' produced by the ovaries during the childbearing years and serves to regulate the menstrual cycle.

Exercise stress test. An electrocardiogram used to measure heart rate and its electrical activity while the participant exercises on a treadmill or stationary bike. The test is used to detect advanced coronary artery disease prior to starting an exercise program.

Free Radicals. Unpaired electrons that forms in the body from normal metabolism, inflammation, stress, and other factors. These unpaired electrons circulate in the body looking for "partners" with which to pair up (atoms normally exist paired). In their quest for partnership, free radicals damage important cellular structures such as cell membrane and DNA, which can lead to genetic mutation, cancer and other ailments. Antioxidants donate electrons to free radicals, thereby minimizing potential damage and disease.

Glycemic Index. The ranking of carbohydrates on a scale from 0 to 100 based on the extent to which they raise blood sugar levels after consumption.

Heart attack. Also referred to as a myocardial infarction, this event has to do with stoppage of oxygen-rich blood flow to a part of the heart muscle.

Heart rate. Reflected by the pulse, the heart rate refers to the number of times the heart pumps blood per minute.

Herxheimer Reaction. A condition where retained toxins are released faster than the body can jettison them. Signs of a Herxheimer Reaction include headache, nausea, vomiting, and fatigue.

High-density lipoprotein (HDL) cholesterol. The so-called good cholesterol that has been shown to protect against coronary heart disease by removing extra fatty material from the blood vessels.

High blood pressure. See *hypertension.*

Homocysteine. An amino acid, derived from protein, which has been associated with increased risk for heart disease and stroke.

Hormones. Substances secreted by an endocrine gland that influence the activities of various organs (e.g., aldosterone secreted by the adrenal gland helps the kidneys conserve water and salt).

Hypercholesterolemia. A blood cholesterol exceeding the desirable level of 200 mg/dL (dL = deciliter = one-tenth of a liter) in both men and women.

Hypertension. Abnormally high blood pressure within the blood vessels caused by increased volume of circulating blood and/or decreased diameter of the blood vessels, among other factors. Hypertension and high blood pressure are interchangeable terms.

Hypoglycemia. Low blood sugar.

Hypotension. Low blood pressure defined as blood pressure below 100/60.

Kidneys. Bean-shaped organs that detoxify the body by removing poisonous waste products. The kidneys also regulate electrolyte, acid–base, water, and salt balance in the body.

Leaky gut syndrome. A condition in which undigested protein seep through the intestinal wall into the blood stream, creating an allergic reaction.

Low-density lipoprotein (LDL) cholesterol. The so-called bad cholesterol that has been shown to cause coronary heart disease by accumulating within the blood vessel walls.

Lipid profile. A blood test that measures the levels of the various fats in the blood.

Lipids. A name for various fats found in the body that include cholesterol and triglycerides.

Lipoproteins. The complex of cholesterol and fat joined with protein carriers. The types of lipoproteins are high-density lipoproteins (HDL), low-density lipoproteins (LDL), and very low density lipoproteins (VLDL).

Low blood pressure. See *hypotension.*

Magnesium. A metallic element that is crucial to the function of bones, muscles, nerves, and other bodily tissues.

Magnetic resonance imaging (MRI). Highly specialized imaging technique that uses magnets and computers to form a three-dimensional image of internal organs.

Metabolic syndrome. The convergence of multiple risk factors that place a person at risk for heart disease, stroke, and cancer. These factors include: a low high-density lipoprotein (HDL or so-called "good") cholesterol; high triglycerides level; mildly elevated blood pressure; and a tendency to gain weight around the waist.

Myocardial infarction. Also called a heart attack, it refers to infarction (death) of heart muscle cells.

Neurotransmitters. A list of chemicals present in the brain and elsewhere that help relay information between nerve cells. Dopamine, serotonin and other neurotransmitters carry messages throughout the network of brain cells.

Nurse practitioner. A registered nurse with advanced training to perform many health care tasks traditionally provided by a physician.

Nutrient-dense. Nutrient dense foods are those packing the most vitamins, minerals, macronutrients, phytochemicals, and fiber for the fewest number of calories. This means fresh, high-quality, organic, unprocessed, whole foods.

Obesity. Defined as 20 percent to 30 percent over ideal body weight. See body mass index chart in Appendix IV.

Organic Foods. Foods produced without using conventional pesticides, synthetic fertilizers, sewage sludge, or ionizing radiation. Organic meats, poultry, eggs and dairy products come from animals that are given no antibiotic or growth hormones.

Osteoporosis. The thinning of the bones that places them at risk for fractures. Both men and women are at risk for osteoporosis, but a drop in estrogen levels during perimenopause and menopause impose a higher risk to women. The best way to treat osteoporosis is to prevent it by pursuing daily weight-bearing exercises and by consuming the proper amounts of calcium, vitamin D, and magnesium.

Palpate. The act of feeling with the hands, as when, for example, a physician feels for the consistency and size of a mass in the abdomen.

Parasympathetic nervous system. See *autonomic nervous system.*

PA. See *physician assistant.*

Percuss. The act of tapping, as when, for example, a physician taps over the liver to determine its size. Percussion uses the physical characteristics of various body structures—e.g., tapping over the liver produces a dull sound—to decide if abnormalities exist.

Physician assistant (PA). A health care professional who, by formal training and experience, performs many medical functions traditionally performed by a physician. Studies have shown that primary care PAs typically carry out 80 percent to 90 percent of tasks performed by general practice physicians.

Phytonutrients. A long list of nutrients derived from plants. These nutrients impart tremendous health benefits, most of which are still being defined.

Plaque. Fatty deposits in the blood vessels that reduce the free flow of blood.

Potassium. A vital electrolyte found in the blood and cells that plays a key role in the function of nerves and muscles, including the heart muscle. Potassium can be found in foods such as orange juice and bananas.

Primary hypertension. The most common of the two types of high blood pressure, the causes of primary hypertension are unknown, but there are risk factors known to contribute to its causation. Also referred to as essential hypertension, this form of hypertension occurs in 90% of persons with high blood pressure.

Probiotics. Live, microbial cultures containing gut-friendly bacteria such as lactobacillus and bifidobacterium.

Prognosis. A prediction regarding the expected course of a disease process.

Refined grains. Foods made from grains that have been milled, which removes the bran and germ along with fiber, iron, and the B vitamins. On the other hand, whole grains are foods made from the entire grain seed (i.e., the kernel), which is made up of the endosperm, germ, and bran.

Risk factor. A condition and or habit that incurs increased likelihood of developing a disease. Obesity, smoking, high alcohol intake, and excessive sodium consumption are among the most prevalent risk factors for high blood pressure.

Salt. A crystallized form of sodium chloride. Sodium causes fluid retention and elevated blood pressure.

Saturated fat. A fatty acid that is "saturated" with hydrogen atoms and thus cannot combine with any more hydrogen. Solid at room temperature, this fat is found in cheese, butter, red meat, and eggs, among other foods. Saturated fats have been shown to raise blood cholesterol levels.

Sleep apnea. Transient stoppage of breathing while asleep. Its causes include obesity, and it can lead to high blood pressure.

Sodium. A mineral element that, in the body, controls water balance, nerve impulse, muscle contraction, and acid–base balance. Approximately 40% of table salt (chemical name, sodium chloride) is sodium. People who are salt sensitive run the risk of developing high blood pressure if they take in large quantities of sodium.

Sphygmomanometer. Also referred to as a blood pressure cuff, this device is used to measure blood pressure.

Stethoscope. An instrument used to listen to various bodily noises such as the heart beat, lung sounds, and arterial sounds.

Stress. The response to perceived threat to our psychological or physical well–being, and the realization that we lack the resources necessary to cope with that threat.

Stroke. Also referred to as cerebrovascular accident, or CVA. Stroke is a sudden loss of function of a part of the brain due to cessation of blood flow caused by a blood vessel rupture (hemorrhage) or blockage (by a clot). Strokes can lead to paralysis and death. Hypertension is the most important risk factor for stroke.

Systolic blood pressure. The top number of a person's blood pressure that reflects the pressure within the arteries when the heart contracts. If a person's blood pressure is 118/66, his or her systolic blood pressure is 118.

Trans-fat. A manufactured fat in which hydrogen is added to vegetable oil—a process called hydrogenation—used to increase the shelf life and flavor of foods. Trans fats can be found in many foods such as margarine, vegetable shortenings, cookies, snack foods, and microwave popcorn. Like saturated fats, trans fats raise total and LDL cholesterol and lowers HDL cholesterol, increasing your risk for heart disease and stroke.

Triglycerides. One of the various types of fat that circulates in the blood and is used for energy or stored in the body as fat. Triglycerides are manufactured in the liver or obtained from dietary sources.

Unsaturated fats. Liquid at room temperature, these fats are found in corn, sunflower and other vegetable oils. Unsaturated fats help lower blood cholesterol levels.

Vascular. Refers to blood vessels (arteries, veins, arterioles, capillaries).

Veins. Blood vessels that carry blood from the body back to the heart for oxygen replenishment.

Wellness. A way of living that emphasizes preventive health strategies such as regular physical activity, healthy nutrition, quality sleep, stress management, and periodic health check-ups.

Whole grains. Foods made from the entire grain seed (i.e., the kernel), which is made up of the endosperm, germ, and bran. On the other hand, refined grains have been milled, which removes the bran and germ along with fiber, iron, and the B vitamins.

Xenoestrogens. Novel, man-made compounds that occupy estrogen receptors in the body because their chemical structures mimic naturally-occurring estrogen.

X-ray. The use of high-energy beams of electrons to image bones and other body parts.

Appendix I

Health and Wellness Resources

American Diabetic Association
www.diabetes.org

American Heart Association
www.americanheart.org

American Lung Association
www.lungusa.org

National Cancer Institute
www.cancer.gov

National Institute on Aging
www.nia.nid.gov

National Sleep Foundation
1522 K Street, NW, Suite 500
Washington, D.C. 20005
www.sleepfoundation.org

Natural Products Association
1773 T Street, NW
Washington, DC 20009
Ph: (202) 223-0101
Fax: (202) 223-0250
E-mail: natural@naturalproductsassoc.org
URL: http://www.naturalproductsassoc.org

Office of the Surgeon General
5600 Fishers Lane
Room 18-66
Rockville, MD 20857
Ph: (301) 443-4000
Fax: (301) 443-3574
URL: http://www.surgeongeneral.gov

Detoxification Programs

(1) The Milis Detoxification Program
http://www.milis.com/pdf/detoxification_program/pdf

(2) Dr. Michael Lam's Detoxification Program
http://www.drlam.com

Hair Mineral Analysis

(1) Bio-Trend Technologies
PO Box 497
Lambertville, MI 48144
http://www.eidon.com/hair_analysis.htm

Appendix II
Suggested Reading

A. Weil. *Healthy Aging: A Lifelong Guide to Your Physical and Spiritual Well-Being.* New York, NY: Anchor Books: 2007

B. J. Willcox, D. C. Willcox and M. Suzuki. *The Okinawa Diet Plan.* New York: Clarkson Potter: 2004.

D. Buettner. *The Blue Zones.* Washington, D.C: The National Geographic Society: 2008.

M. Pollan. *In Defense of Food: An Eater's Manifesto.* New York, NY: Penguin Books, 2008.

M. Hyman and M. Liponis. *Ultraprevention.* New York, NY: Atria Books, 2003.

Appendix III

Food and Exercise Log

Time of Day	Food eaten	Carbohydrates (Calories)	Protein (calories)	Fat (Calories)	Exercise performed (Type & duration)
6:00-7:00 AM (Breakfast)					
10:00 AM (Snack)					
12:00 AM (Lunch)					
3:00 PM (Snack)					
5:00 PM (Dinner)					
8:00 PM (Snack)					

Appendix IV

Body Mass Index Chart

	120	130	140	150	160	170	180	190	200	210	220	230	240	250
4'6	29	31	34	36	39	41	43	46	48	51	53	56	58	60
4'8	27	29	31	34	36	38	40	43	45	47	49	52	54	56
4'10	25	27	29	31	34	36	38	40	42	44	46	48	50	52
5'0	23	25	27	29	31	33	35	37	39	41	43	45	47	49
5'2	22	24	26	27	29	31	33	35	37	38	40	42	44	46
5'4	21	22	24	26	28	29	31	33	34	36	38	40	41	43
5'6	19	21	23	24	26	27	29	31	32	34	36	37	39	40
5'8	18	20	21	23	24	26	27	29	30	32	34	35	37	38
5'10	17	19	20	22	23	24	26	27	29	30	32	33	35	36
6'0	16	18	19	20	22	23	24	26	27	28	30	31	33	34
6'2	15	17	18	19	21	22	23	24	26	27	28	30	31	32
6'4	15	16	17	18	20	21	22	23	24	26	27	28	29	30
6'6	14	15	16	17	19	20	21	22	23	24	25	27	28	29
6'8	13	14	15	17	18	19	20	21	22	23	24	25	26	28

Healthy Weight · Overweight · Obese

$$\text{BMI}= \left\{\frac{\text{WEIGHT (pounds)}}{\text{HEIGHT (inches)}}\right\} \times 703$$

BMI	Weight Status
Below 18.5	Underweight
18.5-24.9	Normal
25.0-29.9	Overweight
30.0 and Above	Obese

Index